Teaching Strategies for Improving Youth Fitness

Second Edition

Robert P. Pangrazi
Charles B. Corbin

Printed in the United States of America
Second Edition

Editors: Nancy Rosenberg and Cathy Kreyche
Design and layout: Jeffrey Biggs
Illustrations: Bruce W. Peschel
Director of Publications: Debra Lewin

ISBN 0-88314-566-9

Contents

1 All About The Prudential FITNESSGRAM

2 Preparing for The Prudential FITNESSGRAM Test

3 Administration of The Prudential FITNESSGRAM Test

4 After Testing: The Physical Fitness Program

Fitness Activities for Primary Grade Students

Fitness Activities for Intermediate-Grade Students

6 Family Fitness Activities

Suggested Presentations

7 Resource Materials

8 Visual Aids and Handouts

Foreword

On December 18, 1993, a partnership agreement was signed by the American Alliance for Health, Physical Education, Recreation and Dance (AAHPERD) and the Cooper Institute for Aerobics Research (CIAR) to promote health-related youth fitness. This partnership unites two of the foremost leaders in the field of health and fitness.

Under the terms of the agreement, AAHPERD will develop and produce fitness education materials and CIAR will develop the fitness assessment and supporting materials. Thus, this second edition of *Teaching Strategies for Improving Youth Fitness*, previously published by CIAR, is published by AAHPERD. Both organizations wish to thank the authors, Dr. Robert Pangrazi and Dr. Charles Corbin, for their continued support of health-related youth fitness, as evidenced by their willingness to produce this book and serve on advisory committees for our joint programs. They are both very esteemed authors and workshop facilitators in the physical education arena. We are proud to have them associated with our programs.

—A. Gilson Brown
Executive Vice President, AAHPERD

—Charles Sterling
Executive Director, CIAR

Preface

This second edition of *Teaching Strategies for Improving Youth Fitness* is revised to make the activities and materials compatible with the new Prudential FITNESSGRAM. The Prudential FITNESSGRAM includes a scientifically based test battery, a new Prudential FITNESSGRAM report card, and state-of-the-art software for generating fitness reports and keeping records.

This handbook was developed to provide fitness ideas and activities to complement the other Prudential FITNESSGRAM materials. It is for teachers, parents, scout leaders, recreation leaders, and any others interested in youth fitness. As the reader can see, it uses school examples because many youth fitness programs are school based. However, the philosophies, programs, tests, and other materials described in this manual can be adapted to a variety of situations.

Teaching Strategies for Improving Youth Fitness is based on the idea that to improve fitness among youth we need more than periodic fitness testing. A good fitness program can be organized around a good fitness test, a sound recognition program, and a fitness report card. However, The Prudential FITNESSGRAM is more. The Prudential FITNESSGRAM System as outlined in this manual includes a philosophy, a multitude of activities, and suggestions of all kinds. Fundamental to fitness development are the notions that "Fitness is for everyone" and that "Fitness is fun." We hope that you use this book to ensure that all youth have an opportunity to develop fitness and to *enjoy both exercise and fitness.*

The Prudential FITNESSGRAM System is not meant to be a substitute for school physical education. It could be an important part of a good physical education program, or it could be in addition to a good program. Properly conducted, The Prudential FITNESSGRAM System will involve all children, their families, and the entire community.

The authors would especially like to thank Marilu Meredith for the many hours of work organizing and editing the manuscript. Thanks also are extended to Margie Ratliff and Bruce Peschel for their work in making the book attractive and easy to read; to Charles Sterling, founder of The Prudential FITNESSGRAM for his continuing efforts on behalf of youth fitness; and to Kenneth Cooper for his continued commitment to the fitness of American youth.

Sharon Plowman and Jim Morrow, both members of The Prudential FITNESSGRAM Advisory Council, are to be thanked for many hours of proofreading and suggestions. Thanks also to Steve Blair, Kirk Cureton, Harold Falls, Tim Lohman, Jim Sallis, Jo Safrit, and Russ Pate, also members of the Advisory Council, for their suggestions. Without the commitment of The Prudential FITNESSGRAM Advisory Council, The Prudential FITNESSGRAM would not have developed into the total fitness system that it has become. Few people are aware of the many hours that these people have given, free of charge, to benefit the youth of our nation.

Finally, we would like to thank the Cooper Institute for Aerobics Research for developing The Prudential FITNESSGRAM and to The Prudential for sponsoring this important project. These two groups have provided the development and sponsorship of The Prudential FITNESSGRAM and all of its components. As a result of their efforts, millions of youth have benefitted.

—Robert P. Pangrazi and Charles B. Corbin

Introduction

Teaching Strategies for Improving Youth Fitness is a timely curriculum manual for use by all fitness leaders who are using The Prudential FITNESSGRAM System. The manual was written to suggest effective strategies for use in implementing a youth fitness program which emphasizes the development of exercise behavior rather than high level fitness performance.

The Prudential FITNESSGRAM System was developed by The Cooper Institute for Aerobics Research. The Prudential Insurance Company, America's largest insurance company, is the exclusive sponsor of FITNESSGRAM. The philosophy, assessment, and recognition program have been further refined by the FITNESSGRAM Advisory Council. This group of respected leaders in the physical education and physical fitness profession, responding to a need for a new approach to solving the problems of youth fitness, have shaped FITNESSGRAM into a total system. which is an outgrowth of the philosophy introduced in my first book Aerobics, published in 1968.

The strategies provided by noted authors Robert Pangrazi and Charles Corbin were selected primarily for their effectiveness in "educating" children about physical fitness and the importance of regular activity. Implementing The Prudential FITNESSGRAM system philosophy is more than conducting fitness activities, it requires the development of a total learning environment which recognizes the importance of the individual and the ability of each person to be responsible for directing his/her personal fitness program. Adopting such a philosophy is perhaps the only way to ensure that a program will provide the "fitness education" necessary for a child to reach the top of the Stairway to Lifetime Fitness and become a wise fitness consumer.

I have been pleased during the last twenty-five years to see that Americans are progressing in their battle against heart disease. However, I am also painfully aware, that all of this progress can be wiped out if children and youth do not join in the battle by staying or becoming regularly active, following prudent nutritional guidelines, and avoiding cigarette smoking. *Teaching Strategies for Improving Youth Fitness* can help you help your students achieve the most important objective, a fitness lifestyle.

—Kenneth H. Cooper, M.D., M.P.H.

— 1 —

All About The Prudential FITNESSGRAM

The Prudential FITNESSGRAM is a complete fitness and exercise program for school-age students and youth. The principal goal of The Prudential FITNESSGRAM is to provide an educational fitness and exercise program that will promote lifetime health-related fitness.

The Prudential FITNESSGRAM Philosophy

The Prudential FITNESSGRAM philosophy is based on three basic assumptions. These assumptions are:

◆ Exercise and fitness are for all people, regardless of gender, age, ability, disability, or any other factor.
◆ Exercise and fitness are for a lifetime.
◆ Doing regular exercise and getting fit can, and should be, fun and enjoyable.

Given these basic assumptions, The Prudential FITNESSGRAM is based on the belief that if people "give effort" and follow basic exercise principles, their fitness will improve. The program encourages regular activity for all people. Recognition is given to those who do regular exercise, because regular exercise will lead to good health and fitness. A report card provides the student and parent with information and suggestions for behavior that will lead to future improvement. Recognition is designed to give people reinforcement that they are "doing the right behavior," to reward their effort and regular physical activity, and to provide information showing they are competent and healthy. The accompanying exercise programs are fun, but challenging. They are designed to instill the notion that exercise is enjoyable.

The Objectives of The Prudential FITNESSGRAM

The Prudential FITNESSGRAM, and all of its educational components, has the following specific objectives:

◆ To stimulate students to be intrinsically motivated to be physically active for a lifetime.
◆ To stimulate students to be intrinsically motivated to be fit for a lifetime.
◆ To provide sound evaluation procedures to test the health-related fitness of school-age students.
◆ To provide health standards to help students, parents, and teachers determine fitness areas in need of improvement.
◆ To provide information to students, parents, and teachers concerning the health-related fitness of those tested.
◆ To teach students important facts and concepts of exercise and fitness.
◆ To provide educationally sound information for improving the exercise behaviors and fitness levels of students.
◆ To provide a recognition program that will promote the previously stated objectives.

The Prudential FITNESSGRAM Program Components

The three major components of The Prudential FITNESSGRAM are the fitness assessment, the report card and computer program, and the recognition program. Each component is described in more detail on the following pages.

The Prudential FITNESSGRAM Assessment

The Prudential FITNESSGRAM assessment measures three components of physical fitness which have been identified as being important because of their relationship to overall health and optimal functioning. The three components are aerobic capacity, body composition, and muscle fitness (strength, endurance, and flexibility). Several test options are provided for each area with one test item being recommended. (Asterisks indicate the tests that are recommended and that are used as the default on the software available with The Prudential FITNESSGRAM program.)

Aerobic Capacity

Teachers will select one of the following options.
- **One Mile Run/Walk**
- **The PACER**—recommended for grades K–3 (multi-stage 20-meter shuttle run)

Body Composition

Teachers will select one of the following options.
- **Percent Fat**—calculated from triceps and calf skinfolds
- **Body Mass Index**—calculated from height and weight

Muscle Fitness (Strength, Endurance, and Flexibility)

Teachers will select as indicated:

Abdominal Strength
Must select.
- Curl-up*

Trunk Extensor Strength and Flexibility
Must select.
- Trunk Lift*

Upper Body Strength
Select one.
- Push-up*
- Modified Pull-up
- Pull-up
- Flexed-Arm Hang

Flexibility
Select one.
- Back-saver Sit-and-Reach*
- Shoulder Stretch

The Prudential FITNESSGRAM Report Card

The report card (see VA 1.1) is designed to give students, teachers, and parents a report of fitness test results. It can be done on a computer or by hand. It reports fitness test results and indicates the extent to which students meet good health criteria.

Features of The Prudential FITNESSGRAM Report Card
The Prudential FITNESSGRAM report card has numerous special features as listed below.
1. Provides highly personalized output.
2. Indicates current and past test performance.
3. Provides individualized exercise recommendations are based on assessment results.
4. Evaluates performance based on criterion-referenced health standards. Scores are classified as Needs Improvement, in the Healthy Fitness Zone, or above the Healthy Fitness Zone.
5. Includes a bar graph of current assessment results.
6. Provides an estimated VO_2max adjusted according to kilogram of body weight per minute to allow comparison between performances on alternative test items.
7. Reports changes in height and weight.

The Prudential FITNESSGRAM Recognition Program

"It's Your Move" is the primary Prudential FITNESSGRAM recognition program and is designed to motivate students to be active and to want to take fitness tests. Other components of the recognition program are:
◆ Get Fit
◆ The Prudential FITNESSGRAM Honor Recognition
◆ I'm Fit
◆ Fit for Life
◆ The Local Recognition Certificate

The Purpose of This Book

This book is designed to help teachers, parents, and those interested in promoting fitness among students. It includes materials to supplement the information presented in The Prudential FITNESSGRAM *Test Administration Manual*. The Prudential FITNESSGRAM is meant to be more than a test that is done in the fall and spring with nothing in between. A quality program should be continuous. It should follow good exercise principles and ideally be part of a total program of physical education. Figure 1 indicates steps that should be included in a quality fitness program. Information included in this book will help you accomplish these steps.

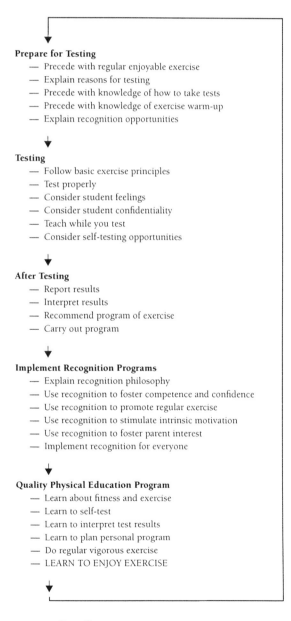

Prepare for Testing
— Precede with regular enjoyable exercise
— Explain reasons for testing
— Precede with knowledge of how to take tests
— Precede with knowledge of exercise warm-up
— Explain recognition opportunities

Testing
— Follow basic exercise principles
— Test properly
— Consider student feelings
— Consider student confidentiality
— Teach while you test
— Consider self-testing opportunities

After Testing
— Report results
— Interpret results
— Recommend program of exercise
— Carry out program

Implement Recognition Programs
— Explain recognition philosophy
— Use recognition to foster competence and confidence
— Use recognition to promote regular exercise
— Use recognition to stimulate intrinsic motivation
— Use recognition to foster parent interest
— Implement recognition for everyone

Quality Physical Education Program
— Learn about fitness and exercise
— Learn to self-test
— Learn to interpret test results
— Learn to plan personal program
— Do regular vigorous exercise
— LEARN TO ENJOY EXERCISE

Figure 1. Steps to a quality fitness program.

How to Use This Book

In the following chapters, many materials are provided to supplement the basic Prudential FITNESSGRAM program. Chapter 2 describes a multitude of pretest activities for students. Included are techniques for preparing students to take The Prudential FITNESSGRAM assessment. The activities described in this chapter should be done before students take The Prudential FITNESSGRAM test.

Chapter 3 is devoted to suggestions for administering The Prudential FITNESSGRAM test, including testing objectives, practical suggestions for administering each test, suggestions for preparing The Prudential FITNESSGRAM report cards, and many other useful tips. Chapter 4 presents activities that can be used between tests. Included are physical activities that can be done to improve fitness as well as ideas for teaching important fitness concepts.

Chapter 5 includes suggestions for implementing the recognition program, and chapter 6 includes suggestions for involving the entire family in fitness activities. Chapter 7 presents information about various resource materials that can help you in building a quality fitness program.

Finally, chapter 8 includes 58 blackline masters that can be duplicated to make visual aids, take-home handouts, or in-class resource materials. These blackline masters will be referred to as visual aids and will be abbreviated with the letters VA. Each visual aid is given a number (relating to a chapter) so that it can be easily located. Throughout the book the reader is referred to different visual aids and how they can be used. For more details, refer to chapter 8.

~ 2 ~

Preparing for The Prudential FITNESSGRAM Test

Before the administration of The Prudential FITNESSGRAM test (or any fitness test), students should be prepared to take the test. Suggestions for preparing students to take The Prudential FITNESSGRAM test are presented in this chapter. Materials are not divided based on the grade level of the students. For this reason, you may have to adapt some of the information to suit the age and developmental level of your students. In general, it is felt that these materials, with proper adaptation, can be used for students at any level.

Teach the Meaning of Fitness

For a program of fitness to be effective, it is important that students know the definition of fitness. Discuss the meaning of total fitness and describe the five different areas of fitness. Visual aids (VA 2.1 and VA 2.2 in chapter 8) can be used to teach the meaning of each area of fitness. It is important to inform students that everyone can improve the different areas of health-related fitness with regular exercise and that improvement in these fitness areas has been shown to reduce the risk of health problems and injury for adults. Students should also understand that although an active lifestyle and fitness are invest-ments in a healthy adult life, activity and fitness can also be important in their daily lives. Benefits include being healthy, looking good, feeling good, and having adequate energy to enjoy all aspects of busy lives. Fitness level may also impact their ability to participate successfully in recreational and competitive sports and other physical activities. Teaching points are listed below.

Total Fitness Allows a Person to:

◆ **Meet emergencies**—Run for help when a friend has been hurt, climbing over fences or jumping a creek if necessary.
◆ **Be healthy**—Reduce the risk of diseases such as heart disease, back prob-lems, obesity, diabetes, and so on.
◆ **Work efficiently**—Work with less fatigue and with more efficiency.
◆ **Enjoy leisure**—Have energy to do physical activities, such as playing sports, during free time.
◆ **Look good**—Look your best by building muscles and maintaining a desir-able level of body fat (not too much and not too little).
  (Adapted from C. B. Corbin and R. Lindsey, *Fitness for Life*, 3rd ed., Glenview, IL: Scott, Foresman and Co., 1990, used by permission.)

The Areas of Health-Related Physical Fitness Are:

◆ **Aerobic capacity**—The ability to exercise the total body for a long period of time without stopping. It requires a fit and healthy heart muscle, blood vessels, and lungs.
◆ **Muscular strength**—The amount of force muscles can produce. It is often measured by how much weight can be lifted.
◆ **Muscular endurance**— The ability of each different group of muscles to do an activity many times without getting tired.
◆ **Flexibility**—The ability to use joints fully. Muscles and joint connective tissue should be stretched regularly to prevent stiffness and a reduction in the range of motion.
◆ **Body composition**—The percent of total body weight that is fat as differ-entiated from lean muscle, bones, and fluid. A person does not want too much or too little of the body to be fat.
  (Adapted from C. B. Corbin and R. Lindsey, *Fitness for Life*, 3rd ed., Glenview, IL: Scott, Foresman and Co., 1990, used by permission.)

Explain the Reasons for Testing

Students should be motivated to give their best performance for testing to be meaningful. One way to motivate students is to inform them of the reasons for testing. VA 2.3 can be used to help students understand why they are being tested. Explain each of the points and allow the students to discuss each point, as well as ask questions. Basic points are listed below.

◆ **Acceptable health fitness standards**—Achieving fitness scores in the Healthy Fitness Zone may help reduce the risk of health problems.
◆ **Need for improvement**—Test results will help the student know personal strengths and weaknesses. The areas needing improvement can be seen.
◆ **Fitness changes**—Test results can be used to see if fitness level has improved or decreased over time. Students may self-test any time they wish to know if they are making progress in their fitness program.
◆ **Benefits**—Good fitness and regular exercise can help students **be healthy, look good, feel good, and enjoy life**. It can help in school work and in playing sports.

Explain the Meaning of Criterion-Referenced Standards

Many students are used to having test results reported in percentiles. They may have previously learned that their physical fitness depends upon how they compare to other people of the same age and sex. Unfortunately, a student may also think "I am a failure" if he or she scores too low to receive a good grade or to earn a fitness award. This can occur even when a student has achieved a very good fitness score (for example, a 75th percentile is a very good percentile score but may not earn a good grade or a fitness award). Since the goal of The Prudential FITNESSGRAM is to promote exercise and fitness for a lifetime, not just for now, the use of comparative standards such as percentiles is discouraged when reporting test results to individual students.

Instead, criterion-referenced standards are used. These standards (established by leading fitness experts) are based on levels of fitness necessary for good health. **IT IS VERY IMPORTANT for students to realize that achieving minimal or acceptable standards of fitness is important to good health.** VA 2.4 may be used to show problems of low fitness.

Specifically, you can explain that low-level aerobic capacity results in increased risk of heart disease, including arteriosclerosis (deposits on the wall of the artery), stroke, heart attack, and high blood pressure. If strength, muscular endurance, and flexibility are poor, there is a greater than normal risk of back problems, muscle soreness, muscle injury, and poor posture. Very high levels of body fat increase the risk of heart disease and other illnesses such as diabetes. Being "overfat" may also cause teenagers numerous psychological problems related to poor self-concept and peer acceptance. A level of body fat that is too low may indicate the presence of an eating disorder such as bulimia or anorexia nervosa, or it may only indicate that the student is exceptionally lean. It should be emphasized that too low a level of body fat can be as dangerous to health as too high a level.

To help students, teachers, and parents interpret test results, The Prudential FITNESSGRAM classifies performance in two general areas: **Needs Improvement** and **Healthy Fitness Zone.** All students should strive to achieve a score that places them inside the Healthy Fitness Zone. It is possible for some students to score above the Healthy Fitness Zone. The Prudential FITNESSGRAM acknowledges performances above the Healthy Fitness Zone but does not recommend this level of performance as an appropriate goal level for all students. Students who desire to achieve a high level of athletic performance may need to consider setting goals that are beyond the Healthy Fitness Zone. Students, especially younger students, may need assistance in setting realistic goals. **The most important objective is to achieve fitness scores in the Healthy Fitness Zone and to do the best you can.**

Healthy Fitness Zone

Needs Improvement	Good	Better

Current research findings were used as the basis for establishing The Prudential FITNESSGRAM health fitness standards. Steven Blair and his colleagues reported that a significant decrease in risk of all-cause mortality results from getting out of the lower 20 percent of the population with regard to aerobic fitness level (see Footnote 1). They also reported that risk level continues to decrease as fitness levels increase but not as dramatically as simply getting out of the bottom 20 percent. Aerobic capacity standards for the Healthy Fitness

---

1. S. N. Blair, H. O. Kohl III, R. S. Paffenberger, Jr., D. G. Clark, K. H. Cooper, and F. W. Gibbons, Physical fitness and all-cause mortality: A prospective study of healthy men and women, *Journal of the American Medical Association, 262,* 1989, pp. 2395–2401.

Zone have been established so that the lower end of the Healthy Fitness Zone corresponds closely to a fitness level equal to getting out of the lower 20 percent of the population. The upper end of the Healthy Fitness Zone corresponds to a fitness level that would include up to 60 percent of the population.

Percent fat is calculated from equations reported by Mary Slaughter and her colleagues (see Footnote 1). Detailed information on the development of these equations and other issues related to the measurement and interpretation of body composition information is available in *Advances in Body Composition Assessment* (see Footnote 2). Williams and his colleagues reported that students with body fat levels above 25 percent for boys and 30–35 percent for girls are more likely to exhibit elevated cholesterol levels and hypertension (see Footnote 3). The beginning of the Healthy Fitness Zone corresponds to these levels of body fat.

Little or no data exist to indicate levels of musculoskeletal fitness associated with good health. Standards in this area of fitness were established to correspond in level as closely as possible to those in aerobic capacity and body composition.

In interpreting performance on physical fitness assessments, it is most important to remember the following:

◆ The physical fitness experience should always be fun and enjoyable.
◆ Physical fitness testing should not become a competitive sport.
◆ One student's performance should not be compared to that of another student.
◆ The primary reason for testing is to provide the student with personal information that may be used in planning a personal fitness program.
◆ Performance level on fitness tests should not be used as a basis for grading.

Use VA 2.4 to explain that it is important to be in the Healthy Fitness Zone. Beyond that, fitness goals will depend on personal needs and interests. Students who want to play a sport competitively will need to be more fit than

1. M. H. Slaughter, T. G. Johman, R. A. Bodeau, C. A. Horswill, R. J. Stillman, M. D. Van Loan, and D. A. Bemben, Skinfold equations for estimation of body fatness in children and youth, *Human Biology, 60,* 1988, pp. 709–733.

2. T. G. Lohman, *Advances in Body Composition* (Champaign, IL: Human Kinetics Publishers, 1992).

3. P. P. Williams, S. B. Going, D. W. Harsha, L. S. Webber, and G. S. Berenson, Body fatness and the risk of elevated blood pressure, total cholesterol and serum lipoprotein ration in children and youth, *American Journal of Public Health, 82,* 1992, pp. 358–363.

those who do not. Use VA 2.5 and VA 2.6 to discuss the levels of fitness that meet the criteria for good health.

Influence of Body Size and Maturity on Fitness

Body size (height and weight) is to some extent related to physical fitness as measured by a combination of tests. Although there is much variability among individuals, the influence of body size on fitness is especially apparent in two ways:

1. Excess weight associated with fatness tends to have a negative influence on aerobic capacity and on test items in which the body must be lifted or moved (e.g., upper body strength items).
2. Variation in body size associated with maturity can influence fitness around the time of the adolescent growth spurt and sexual maturation. There is considerable variation among individuals in the timing of this maturation period. In adequately nourished students, the timing is largely determined by genetics. Within a given age group of early adolescent students, there will be great variation in the maturation level.

This variation in size and maturity level will influence performance on fitness tests. Boys show a clear growth spurt in muscle mass, strength, power, and endurance and a decrease in subcutaneous fat on the arms and legs. Girls show considerably smaller growth spurts in strength, power, and endurance and tend to accumulate body fat compared to boys. In this age group, students may experience an increase or decrease in their abilities to perform on certain test items completely independent of their levels of physical activity.

In addition to being influenced by maturity, a child's response to training is also determined by genetic background. Some students will improve performance more rapidly than others. Some students will be able to perform at a much higher level than others regardless of training levels.

Precede the Test with Enjoyable Exercise

One of the basic principles of exercise is called the "Principle of Progression." This principle states that exercise should be systematically applied or increased so that a reasonable overload, based on an individual's current fitness level, occurs. Too much exercise too soon will not promote optimal fitness improvement and can cause problems such as soreness, injury, and a dislike for physical activity. For this reason it makes little sense to have students do vigorous exercise on the first day of school. Though some students may be fit as a result of recent regular physical activity, many of them may have been quite inactive during the summer break. Before giving the test, get the students involved in an exercise program. As a general rule, between 2 and 6 weeks should be allowed for students to prepare for fitness testing. Making the exercise fun and enjoyable will help reduce test fear and apprehension. Some specific activities to help get students physically active follow.

Activity 1

Using the Get Fit Exercises

Have the students try each of the exercises in the Get Fit program (VA 2.7). Demonstrate them in class and have the students practice them. Explain the purpose of each exercise. Students should be encouraged to do the exercises at home (for recognition or just to prepare for the test). If not, you may want to use the Get Fit activities in class. Some suggestions for using the Get Fit program are listed below.

- ◆ **Rotate exercise leaders**—Allow students to lead the Get Fit exercises from time to time. As long as the students select exercises listed on the program sheet, allow them to select the exercises to be done. Do the exercises as part of class time and select a different leader each day.
- ◆ **Do the exercises to music.**
- ◆ **Have students create a video**—Use a video recorder with the music and the Get Fit exercises. The video can be used in class for exercise.
- ◆ **Create an exercise circuit using the Get Fit exercises.**
- ◆ **Have the students keep an exercise log and earn the Get Fit recognition**—Rules for earning the recognition are presented on VA 2.8 as well as in The Prudential FITNESSGRAM *Test Administration Manual*. VA 2.8 can be copied and used by students to earn the recognition.

Activity 2

Exercising to Get Ready
for the One Mile Run/Walk or the PACER

The one mile run/walk and the PACER (progressive aerobic cardiovascular endurance run) are measures of aerobic capacity. Students can show improvement in aerobic performance with regular exercise. These test items place demand on the cardiovascular system, which makes it important that students be involved in a number of aerobic activities before participating in them.

Aerobic capacity is genetically limited, and for this reason self-comparison rather than comparison with other students is encouraged. The important factor is that each individual try to accomplish his or her personal best. Students should be involved in activity which lasts for 10 to 15 minutes and raises the heart rate. (Use activity 3 in this chapter to help students learn about target heart rate.) The following are examples of aerobic activities which can be performed daily for several weeks prior to testing. Encourage students to do them with a friend and check their heart rate at regular intervals.

♦ **Walking briskly.**
♦ **Jogging with a friend.**
♦ **The aerobic point system**—Discuss Kenneth Cooper's aerobic point system and encourage students to begin earning aerobic points (see chapter 7).
♦ **Aerobic fitness**—Have students perform an aerobic fitness routine on a regular basis, prior to testing.
♦ **Jumping rope**—Create jump rope routines and mix them with exercises in the Get Fit program.
♦ **Play basketball or soccer.**
♦ **Ride a bicycle.**
♦ **Go hiking.**
♦ **Play active games.**
♦ **Physical education classes**—Physical activity in physical education classes is excellent for preparing for the test, especially if the daily program includes some moderate to vigorous exercise preceded by a warm-up and followed by a cool-down. For some activities, skill development lessons may not be vigorous enough to provide aerobic training benefits, so other vigorous fitness activities will need to be added to the lesson.
♦ **Other activities**—Refer to chapter 4, which contains many other suggestions for developing aerobic capacity.

Activity 3

Learning About Target Heart Rate

To prepare students for fitness testing, they should be involved in physical activity for 2 to 6 weeks prior to the actual testing. It is important that students understand the need to raise the heart rate into the training zone during aerobic activity.

Aerobic fitness benefits occur when students work at 60 percent of their heart rate reserve or higher. The table below is based on the resting heart rate of students. Students should measure their heart rate for a period of 1 to 2 weeks prior to going to bed in the evenings. An average resting heart rate can be recorded and used to determine the range to which their heart rate should be elevated to achieve the training zone. For students, heart rates in excess of 185 usually indicate anaerobic work; thus, for most students 185 can serve as the upper limit of the target zone.

Resting Heart Rate	Target Heart Rate
Below 60	150
60–64	151
65–69	153
70–74	155
75–79	157
80–84	159
85–89	161
90 and over	163

The following activities will assist students in learning about target heart rate:

◆ **Have students complete a chart (VA 2.9) which requires recording their resting heart rate prior to going to bed at night**—For the sake of consistency, it is a good idea to ask them to lie down for 2 or 3 minutes and then measure heart rate for 15 seconds. Each beat should be counted during the 15 seconds and then converted to a 1-minute score by multiplying by four. For example, if the student counts 18 beats in 15 seconds, their heart rate is 72 beats per minute. Younger students may need to ask parents for assistance in doing the multiplication.

◆ **Ask students to develop a target heart rate log (VA 2.10)**—Stipulate different times of the day both in and out of school when they are to take their heart rate. This can be used to stimulate a discussion to illustrate how seldom people move their heart rate into the training zone.

◆ **On different days, try an activity such as rope jumping, walking, jogging, or bicycling to see which elevates the heart rate into the training zone**—Each of the activities should be performed for the same amount of time (5 or 10 minutes) to illustrate that some types of exercise are more demanding than others. The pulse rate should be taken for 6 seconds immediately after cessation of the activity. Record the results on VA 2.11.

◆ **Illustrate how excess body fat impacts the heart rate due to increased workload**—Use two subjects of the same sex who have similar builds, fitness levels, and resting heart rates. Ask one to carry 10 to 15 pounds of extra weight in a backpack. Both students then perform some type of aerobic activity. Immediately take the heart rates at the end of the activity and compare them. Discussion should relate the extra weight being carried in the backpack to excess body fat. This activity can also be done by having one student perform the activity without the backpack and then trying the activity with the backpack.

Activity 4

Aerobic vs. Anaerobic Activities

Cardiovascular exercise can be aerobic or anaerobic. Aerobic activity requires oxygen and can be sustained for long periods of time. Anaerobic metabolism does not require oxygen and provides the body with immediate energy for short bouts of exercise. If aerobic fitness is the desired goal, exercise must be done for a period of time with the heart rate elevated into the target zone (activity 3).

It is important that students understand the difference between the two types of exercise. For health-related fitness, emphasis is placed on aerobic fitness, which is developed by exercise of long duration and moderate intensity. Pacing is important in aerobic activities. Examples of aerobic activities are walking, jogging, swimming, and bicycling. Anaerobic activities are short in duration, usually less than 2 minutes, and quite strenuous. Examples are sprinting, running with the football, and running up the stairs. Anaerobic activities usually require rest upon their completion due to their highly strenuous and demanding nature. The following learning activities should help students understand the differences between aerobic and anaerobic exercise.

♦ **Students need to understand the relationship between duration and intensity**—If the intensity is high, the duration will usually be short. Discuss how running a mile differs from running a sprint. Include the need for pacing in the discussion. Pacing involves moving at a speed that allows the lungs and heart to bring enough oxygen to the muscles for extended activity. It is important that students learn to value aerobic activities for the impact they have on health-related fitness.

♦ **Have students use the worksheet (VA 2.12) that lists a variety of activities and evaluate them in terms of their contribution to aerobic and anaerobic fitness**—Students should personally evaluate each of the activities by trying to perform them. Any activity which students cannot continue for longer than 2 minutes is usually anaerobic in nature. Identify how some anaerobic activities can be modified to make them more aerobic in nature.

♦ **Discuss a number of sports such as football, volleyball, tennis, cross country running, and basketball in terms of anaerobic and aerobic**—Identify which areas of the sport contribute to anaerobic or aerobic fitness. List sports which are better in terms of aerobic fitness.

Activity 5

Increasing Upper-Body Strength and Endurance

Strength is defined as the greatest amount of force a muscle group can exert against a resistance at one time. Endurance is the number of repetitions a muscle group can perform. Most activities require both strength and endurance; thus they are discussed together in this section. Strength and endurance are important requisites in effective skill performance. They are critical in a number of sport skills such as throwing and striking.

To increase strength, it is important that the muscles be required to move the maximum amount of resistance for a few repetitions. On the other hand, a lighter weight moved 10 to 15 repetitions will increase endurance. In the school setting, most activities will cause an increase in both attributes. For example, performing a number of push-ups will increase strength as well as endurance of the triceps muscles. It is important for students to understand that fitness testing will always involve both attributes.

The push-up is the preferred (default) test item for strength and muscular

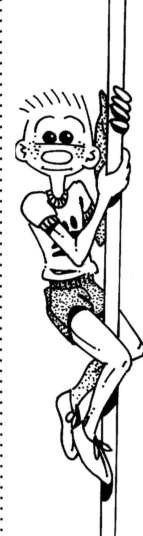

endurance for The Prudential FITNESSGRAM. This item requires strength and endurance primarily in the extensor muscles. Have students perform the following activities to improve on the push-up test.

The push-up demands triceps strength and endurance. The following are challenges that can be done in the regular push-up position to strengthen the triceps muscle group.

◆ Maintain the push-up position and wave at a friend. Wave with the other arm. Shake a leg at someone. Do these challenges in the crab position.
◆ Lift one foot high. Now the other foot.
◆ Inch the feet up to the hands and go back again. Inch the feet up to the hands, and then inch the hands out to return to the push-up position.
◆ Reach up with one hand and touch the other shoulder behind the back.
◆ Turn over so that the back is to the floor. Now complete the turn to push-up position.
◆ Walk on the hands and feet in the push-up position. Try two hands and one foot. Walk in the crab position (tummy toward the ceiling).
◆ Lower the body an inch at a time until the chest touches the floor. Return to the up position any way possible.

All of the exercises listed below develop strength in the flexor muscles. The flexed-arm hang and pull-ups primarily measure the strength and endurance of these muscles. Have students practice these activities.

◆ **Flexed-arm hang**—The flexed-arm hang is used to develop strength in the upper body for students who are not capable of performing a pull-up. Bars should be placed on the playground or between doorjambs at different levels so students can move into place (chin above the bar), lift the knees, and hang.
◆ **Reverse pull-ups**—Students assume the flexed-arm hang position and slowly lower themselves to an extended hanging position. It may be necessary for students to begin on a bar which is lower if they do not have the strength to gradually lower themselves. This will allow them to support part of their weight with the legs and partially lower their body without full arm extension.
◆ **Pole climbing**—Poles such as those used for tetherball can be climbed. For students lacking strength, a box can be placed nearby so they can hang onto the pole and be challenged to stay off the ground as long as possible.
◆ **Rope activities**—There are a number of ways to utilize climbing ropes to develop strength.
   Floor-mounted rope: Students sit on a carpet square and pull them-

selves toward the wall using a rope which is fastened to the wall near floor level. Students can also pull themselves while in a prone position.

Hanging rope with knots: Knots tied in a climbing rope at 12-inch intervals will allow students to grasp the rope more easily. They can also stand on a knot and rest.

Swinging on a rope: Swinging on a climbing rope is suggested since it keeps the body weight supported and is a highly motivating activity. Anytime the arms must support the body weight, arm strength is being developed. Monitor swinging to help prevent falls.

Rope climbing: Students should be encouraged to climb ropes on a regular basis. The focus should be on climbing as high as possible but to a height which allows them to return to the floor using a hand over hand descent.

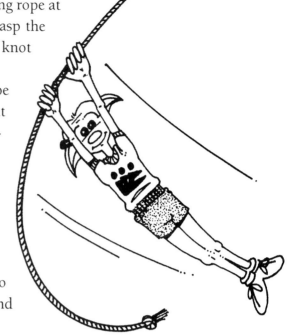

Activity 6

Preparing for the Curl-up Test

Strength and endurance of the abdominal muscles are important for good posture and correct pelvic alignment. Maintaining abdominal strength is important in preventing lower back pain. The curl-up is used as the test item because it does not involve the help of the hip flexor muscles and minimizes compression of the spine (when compared to a full sit-up with the feet held to the floor). It is important that students learn how to develop abdominal strength and endurance using a wide range of fitness challenges. Since it is difficult for some students (particularly primary grade students) to perform curl-up activities, it is necessary to offer some challenges that will teach them to strengthen the abdominals in other ways. The following challenges are lead-up activities that will help develop strength in the abdominal region:

◆ Lift head from the floor and look at the toes. Wink right eye and wiggle the left foot. Reverse.

◆ In a supine position, "wave" a leg at a friend. Use the other leg. Use both legs.

◆ Lift knees up slowly, an inch at a time.

- Curl up any way possible (try pulling on the thighs) and touch right toes with the left hand. Then do it touching left toes with right hand.
- In a sitting position, lean the upper body backward without falling. How long can this position be held?
- From a sitting position, tuck the chin and lower the body slowly to the floor. Vary the positions of the arms (across the tummy, the chest, and above the head).
- From a supine position, hold the shoulders off the floor.
- From a supine position, lift the legs and head off the floor.

Activity 7

Increasing Flexibility

Flexibility can be increased through regular episodes of stretching activity. The sit-and-reach test evaluates the flexibility of the lower back and posterior thighs. This is important since the lack of flexibility in this area is thought to be a factor in the development of lower back pain. Students should understand that degree of flexibility differs just as speed and strength vary among individuals. The important concept is to increase and/or maintain the level of flexibility rather than compare to other individuals.

Students should be taught how to perform static stretches, which are slow and controlled movements. This is in contrast to commonly performed ballistic stretching, which involves rapid bouncing movements. The bouncing movements may cause injury. Static stretches should be made to the point at which the student feels tension in the muscles and be held for 5 to 15 seconds. The legs should not be hyperextended (locked at the knees) when stretches are performed. Perform 3 to 5 repetitions of each stretch. Use the stretching exercises suggested in the Get Fit program or other class favorites to improve flexibility following the guidelines noted above.

Administering The Prudential FITNESSGRAM

On the following pages, descriptions are provided for each of the test items in The Prudential FITNESSGRAM. These descriptions are taken from The Prudential FITNESSGRAM *Test Administration Manual*. For more comprehensive information consult the manual. The following chart summarizes the available test items.

Fitness Component	Test Items	Comment
Aerobic capacity	One mile run/walk[a]	Default test, upper grades
	The PACER	Recommended for grades K–3
Body Composition	Skinfolds[a]	Measures percent fat
	Body mass index	Uses height/weight
Muscle Strength/ Endurance	Curl up[a]	Abdominals
	Push-up[a]	Upper body
	Modified pull-up[b]	Upper body (alternate)
	Pull-up[b]	Upper body (alternate)
	Flexed-arm hang[b]	Upper body (alternate)
	Trunk lift[a]	Trunk extension
Flexibility	Back-saver sit-and-reach[a]	Hip range of motion
	Shoulder stretch	Shoulder range of motion

[a] Item is used as default in software.

[b] For descriptions of these items refer to The Prudential FITNESSGRAM *Test Administration Manual*.

One Mile Run/Walk

Test Objective: The objective is to run and/or walk a one-mile distance at the fastest pace possible. If a student cannot run the total distance, walking is permitted. Performance standards for students in grades K–3 have purposely not been established. The object of the test for these younger students is simply to complete the one-mile distance at a comfortable pace.

Equipment/Facilities: A flat running course, stopwatch, pencil, and scoresheets are required. The course may be a track or any other measured area. The course may be measured using a tape measure or cross country wheel. Caution: If track is metric or shorter than 440 yards, adjust the running course (1,609.34 meters = 1 mile; 400 meters = 437.4 yards; 1,760 yards = 1 mile). On a metric track, add 10 yards to the total 4 laps.

Test Instructions: Students begin on the signal "Ready, Start." As they cross the finish line, elapsed time should be called to the participants (or their partners). It is possible to test 15–20 students at one time by dividing the group and assigning partners. While one group runs, partners count laps and make note of finish time.

Scoring: The one mile run/walk is scored in minutes and seconds. A score of "99" minutes and "99" seconds indicates that the student could not finish the distance. Students in grades K–3 should not be timed; they should simply complete the distance. Enter a score of "0" minutes "0" seconds in the computer if students in grades K–3 complete the one mile.

The PACER

The PACER (progressive aerobic cardiovascular endurance run) is a multistage fitness test adapted from the 20-meter shuttle run test developed in 1982. The test is progressive; it is easy at the beginning and gets harder. Set to music this test can provide a valid, fun alternative to the customary distance run test for measuring aerobic capacity. The PACER is recommended for all ages. Information on music tapes can be obtained by calling (800) 635-7050.

Teachers in grades K–3 are strongly encouraged to use the PACER. When administering the test to these younger students, the emphasis should be to allow the students to have a pleasant, fun experience while learning how to take this test and how to pace. Allow students to continue to run as long as they wish and as long as they are still enjoying the activity. Typically the test in grades K–3 will only last a few minutes. It is not desirable or necessary to make them run to exhaustion.

Test Objective: To run as long as possible back and forth across a 20-meter distance at a specified pace which gets faster each minute.

Equipment/Facilities: A flat, nonslippery surface at least 20 meters in length, cassette player with adequate volume, audio cassette, measuring tape, marker cones, pencil, and scoresheets are required. Students should wear shoes that will prevent slipping. Plan for each student to have a space for running 40–60 inches wide.

Test Instructions: Mark the 20-meter (21 yards and 32 inches) course with marker cones and a tape line or chalk line at each end. Calibrate cassette tape by using the 1-minute test interval at the beginning of the tape. If the tape has stretched and the timing is off more than 0.5 seconds, obtain another copy of the tape. Make copies of the score sheet for each group of students to be tested. The figure on the next page provides diagrams of the testing procedures.

Before test day students should be allowed at least two practice sessions. First allow students to listen to several minutes of the tape so that they know what to expect. Then do a couple of practice runs. Allow students to select a partner. Have students who are being tested line up behind the start line.

The PACER tape has two music versions and one with only the beeps. Each version will give a 5-second countdown (5, 4, 3, 2, 1) and instruct students to "Begin." Students run across the area and touch the line by the time the beep sounds. At the sound of the beep, they turn around and run back to the other end. If some students get to the line before the beep, they must wait for the beep before running the other direction.

Scoring: Have one student record the lap number (crossing off each lap number) on a PACER Wall Chart (provided with PACER test tape). The recorded score is the total **number of laps completed** by the student. The runner's partner should record the total number of times the student reached the line successfully. For students in grades K–3, enter a score of "0" laps to indicate that they successfully completed the PACER run.

When to Stop: Students continue in this manner until they can no longer reach the line before the beep sounds. They reverse directions on the beep (even if they haven't reached the line). Allow a student to attempt to catch up with the pace until he/she has missed two beeps. They are stopped after being unable to reach the line two times (not necessarily in succession). Students who have lost pace should walk from the testing area to a designated cool-down area, being careful not to interfere with others who may still be running. Students just completing the test should continue to walk and stretch in the cool-down area.

Suggestions for Test Administration:
◆ The test tape contains 21 levels (21 minutes). The tape allows 9 seconds to run the distance during the first minute. Each minute the pace increases approximately one-half second.
◆ Single beeps indicate the end of a lap (one 20-meter distance). The student runs from one end to the other between each beep. Triple beeps at the end of each minute indicate the end of a level and an increase in speed. Stu-

dents should be alerted that the speed will increase. **Caution students not to begin too fast.** The beginning speed is very slow. Nine seconds are allowed to run the 20-meter distance during the first minute.

◆ Groups of students may be tested at one time. Adult volunteers may be asked to assist in recording scores.

◆ 40–60 inches of width is required per person for running the test.

Skinfold Measurements

Test Objective: To measure the triceps and calf skinfold thicknesses for calculation of the percent of body fatness.

Equipment/Facilities: A skinfold caliper is necessary to perform this measurement. Costs of calipers range from $5 to $200. Both the expensive and inexpensive calipers have been shown to be effective for use by teachers who have had sufficient training and practice. Chapter 7 includes a listing of possible sources of calipers.

Testing Procedures: The triceps and calf skinfolds have been chosen for The Prudential FITNESSGRAM because they are easily measured and are highly correlated with total body fat. The skinfold fat measure consists of a double layer of subcutaneous fat and skin.

Measurement Locations: The triceps skinfold is measured on the back of the arm over the triceps muscle of the right arm midway between the elbow and the acromion process of the scapula. Using a piece of string to find

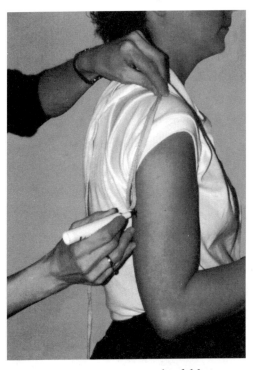
Figure 1. *Locating triceps skinfold site.*

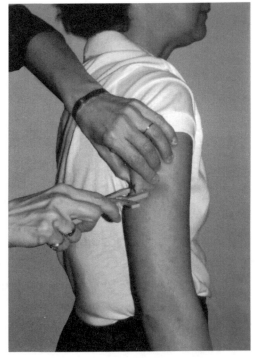
Figure 2. Triceps skinfold measurement.

the midpoint is a good suggestion (see Figure 1). The skinfold site should be vertical. Pinching the fold slightly above the midpoint will ensure that the fold is measured right on the midpoint (see Figures 2).

The calf skinfold is measured on the inside of the right leg at the level of the maximal calf girth. The right foot is placed flat on an elevated surface with the knee flexed at a 90 degree angle (see Figure 3). The vertical skinfold should be grasped just above the level of maximal girth (see Figure 4) and the measurement made below the grasp of maximal girth.

Measurement Technique:
◆ Skinfolds should be measured on the right side of body.
◆ Instruct the student to relax the arm or leg being measured.
◆ Firmly grasp the skinfold between the thumb and forefinger and lift it away from the other body tissue. The grasp should not be so firm as to be painful.
◆ Caliper should be placed in the middle of the fold.
◆ Place caliper ½ inch below the pinch site.
◆ The recommended procedure is to do one measurement at each site before doing the second measurement at each site and finally doing the third set of measurements.

Scoring: The skinfold measure is registered on the dial of the caliper. Each measurement should be taken three times, with the recorded score being the median (middle) of the three scores. To illustrate: if the readings were

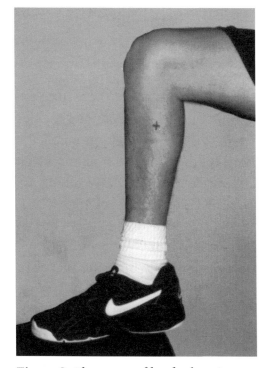

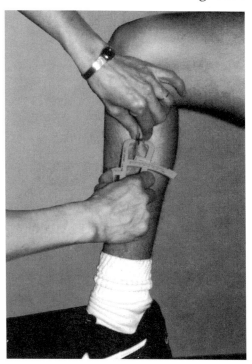

Figure 3. Placement of leg for locating calf skinfold site.

Figure 4. Calf skinfold measurement.

7.0, 8.0, and 9.0, the score would be recorded as 8.0 mm. Each reading should be recorded to the nearest .5 millimeter. Determine percent fat using VA 2.16a and 2.16b.

Suggestions for Test Administration:
◆ Skinfolds should be measured in a setting that provides the student with privacy.
◆ Interpretation of the measurements may be given in a group setting as long as individual results are not identified.
◆ Whenever possible, it is recommended that the same tester administer the skinfold measurement on the same students in subsequent testing periods.
◆ Practice measuring the sites with another tester, and compare results with the same students. As you become familiar with the methods you will find agreement within 10 percent between testers.

Learning to Do Skinfold Measurements:
To learn how to do skinfold measurements, using video training tapes and/or participating in a workshop are excellent ways to begin. The videotape *Measuring Body Fatness Using Skinfolds* illustrates the procedures described in this manual. Chapter 7 contains information on obtaining this videotape.

Body Mass Index

The body mass index provides an indication of the appropriateness of a child's weight relative to height. Body mass index is determined by the following formula:

$$\text{Weight (kg)/Height(m)}^2$$

Height and weight measures recorded as a regular part of the testing process for all students are used by the computer to calculate body mass index. For these calculations, the computer converts weight to kilograms and height to meters. For example, a student weighing 100 pounds and 5 feet in height would have a body mass index of 19.7. Another student also weighing 100 pounds but 5 feet 2 inches tall would have a body mass index of 18.3.

Body mass index is calculated only if skinfold measurements are not entered. Recommended body mass index scores are listed in VA 2.5 and VA 2.6. A score which is classified as Needs Improvement generally indicates that a student weighs too much for his/her height. Body mass index is not the recommended procedure for determining body composition because it does not estimate the percent of fat; it merely provides information on the appropriateness of the weight relative to the height. For those students found to be too heavy for their height, a skinfold test will clarify if the weight is due to excess fat.

Curl-up

Test Objective: To complete as many curl-ups as possible up to a maximum of 75 at a specified pace.

Equipment/Facilities: Gym mats and a cardboard measuring strip for every two students are needed. Two sizes of measuring strips may be needed. The narrower strip is 30 inches x 3 inches and is used to test students in grades K–4; the wider strip is 30 inches x 4½ inches and is used to test older students. Other methods of measuring distance such as using tape strips and pencils are suggested later in this book.

Test Instructions: Allow students to form groups of three. One student will perform the curl-ups, another will place hands under the head of the student doing curl-ups and count, and the third will secure the measuring strip so that it does not move.

The student being tested lies in a supine position on the mat, knees bent at an angle of approximately 140 degrees, **feet flat on the floor**, legs slightly apart, arms straight and parallel to the trunk with palms of hands resting on the mat. The fingers are stretched out and the head is in contact with the partner's hand, resting on the mat.

After the student has assumed the correct position on the mat, place measuring strip under the legs on the mat so that fingertips are just resting on the edge of the measuring strip. The third student in each group should stand astride the one being tested, securing the ends of the measuring strip with the feet (see Figure 5).

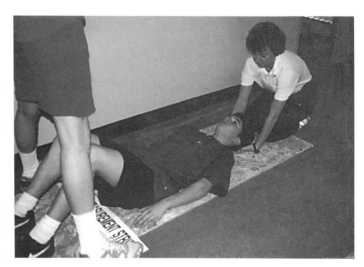

Figure 5. Starting position for the curl-up test.

Keeping heels in contact with the mat, the student curls up slowly, sliding fingers across the measuring strip until fingertips reach the other side (see Figures 6 and 7), then curls back down until the head touches the partner's hand. Movement should be slow and controlled to the specified cadence, which is 20 curl-ups per minute (one curl every 3 seconds). The teacher should call a cadence or use a prerecorded cadence.

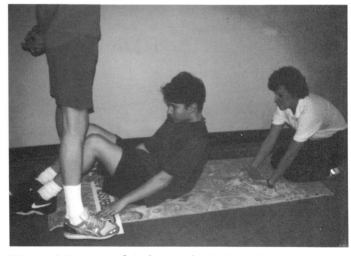

Figure 6. Position of student in the "up" position for the curl-up test.

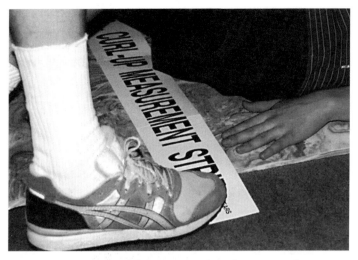

(A recorded cadence may be found on the PACER music tape.) The student continues without pausing until he/she can no longer continue or has completed a maximum number of 75 curl-ups.

When to Stop: Students are stopped after a maximum of 75 curl-ups are completed or two corrections are made. Corrected curl-ups do not count toward the student's score.

Scoring: The score is the number of correctly performed curl-ups. Count should be made when the student's head returns to contact the partner's hand on the mat.

Figure 7. Close-up of fingertips sliding from one side of measuring strip to the other.

Suggestions for Test Administration:
◆ Heels must remain in contact with the mat during the entire curl-up.
◆ The head must contact partner's hands on returning to the floor.
◆ Student must be able to stay with the cadence and not stop to rest.
◆ Movement should start with a flattening of the lower back followed by a slow curling of the upper spine.
◆ The hands should slide across the measuring strip until the fingertips reach the opposite side (3 inches or 4½ inches). Then the student returns to the supine position. The movement is completed when the back of the head touches partner's hand.
◆ The cadence will encourage a steady, continuous movement done in the correct form.

Trunk Lift

It is important that attention is given to performance technique during this test. The movement should be performed in a slow and controlled manner. The maximum score is 12 inches.

Test Objective: To lift the upper body 12 inches off the floor using the muscles of the back and to hold the position to allow for the measurement.

Equipment/Facilities: Gym mats and a flexible rule made of posterboard showing the 6 inch and the 12 inch marks are needed.

Test Description: The student being tested lies on the mat in a prone position (face down). Toes are pointed and hands are placed under the thighs (see Figure 8). The student lifts the upper body off the floor, in a very slow and controlled manner, to a maximum height of 12 inches (see Figure 9). The position is held long enough to allow tester to place the rule on the floor in front of the student and determine the distance of the student's chin from the floor (see Figure 10). The rule should be placed at least an inch to the front of the student's chin and **not directly under the chin**. Once the measurement has been made, the student returns to the starting position in a controlled manner. Allow two trials, recording the highest score.

Scoring: The score is recorded to the nearest inch. Distances above 12 inches should be recorded as 12 inches.

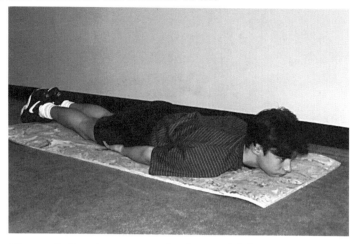

Figure 8. *Starting position for the trunk lift.*

Suggestions for Test Administration:

◆ Do not allow students to do ballistic, bouncing movements.

◆ Do not encourage students to rise higher than 12 inches. The Healthy Fitness Zone ends at 12 inches, and scores beyond 12 inches will not be accepted by the computer. Excessive arching of the back may cause compression of the discs.

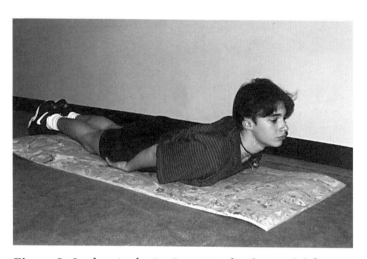

Figure 9. *Student in the "up" position for the trunk lift test.*

Push-up

The push-up to an elbow angle of 90 degrees is the recommended test for upper body strength and endurance. Test administration requires little or no equipment, multiple students may be tested at one time, and few zero scores result. It teaches students an activity that can be used throughout life as a conditioning activity as well as an item for use in self-testing.

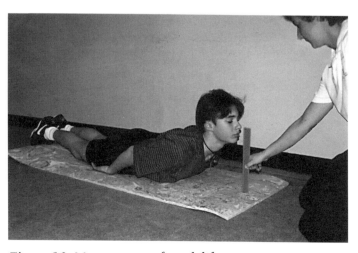

Figure 10. *Measurement of trunk lift.*

Test Objective: To complete as many push-ups as possible at a rhythmic pace.

Equipment/Facilities: The only equipment necessary is an audio cassette with the recorded cadence. The correct cadence is 20 push-ups per minute (one push-up every 3 seconds). The PACER test tape contains a recorded push-up cadence.

Test Instructions: The students should be paired; one will perform the test while the other counts push-ups and watches to see that the student being tested bends the elbow to 90 degrees with the upper arm parallel to the floor.

Prior to test day, students should be allowed to practice doing the push-up and watch their partner do push-ups. Teachers should make an effort during these practice sessions to correct students who are not achieving the 90 degree angle. In this manner, all students will gain greater skill in knowing what 90 degrees "feels like" and "looks like."

The student being tested assumes a prone position on the mat with hands placed under the shoulders; fingers stretched out; legs straight, parallel and slightly apart; and toes tucked under. The student pushes up off the mat with the arms until arms are straight, keeping legs and back straight. The back should be kept in a straight line from head to toes throughout the test (see Figure 11).

The student then lowers the body using the arms until the elbows bend at a 90 degree angle and the upper arms are parallel to the floor (see Figure 12). This movement is repeated as many times as possible. The student should continue the movement until the arms are straight each repetition. The rhythm should be approximately 20 push-ups per minute or 1 push-up every 3 seconds. Cadence should be called or played on a prerecorded tape.

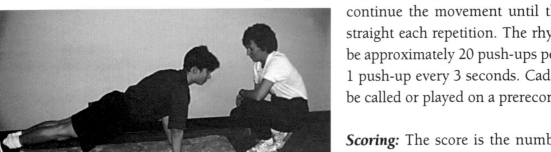

Figure 11. Starting position for push-up test.

Scoring: The score is the number of push-ups completed successfully.

When to stop: Students are stopped after two corrections are made. Corrected push-ups do no count toward the student's score.

◆ Corrections to be monitored are:
    —knees touching floor
    —upper or lower back swaying
    —failing to extend arms fully
    —failing to bend to 90 degrees at the elbow

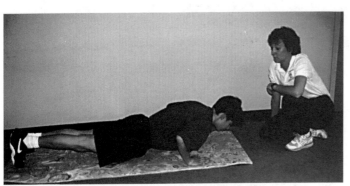

Figure 12. Student in the "down" position for the push-up test.

—jerky movement

—inability to stay with the cadence or stops to rest

The test should be ended if the student appears to be in extreme discomport or pain.

Back-Saver Sit-and-Reach

The back-saver sit-and-reach is very similar to the traditional sit-and-reach except that it is performed on one side at a time. The measurement is performed on one side at a time so that students are not encouraged to hyperextend. The sit-and-reach measures predominantly the flexibility of the hamstring muscles. Normal hamstring flexibility allows rotation of the pelvis in forward bending movements and posterior tilting of the pelvis for proper sitting.

Test Objective: To be able to reach the specified distance on the right and left sides of the body. Distance required to achieve Healthy Fitness Zone is age and sex adjusted and is specified in VA 2.5 and 2.6.

Equipment/Facilities: This assessment requires a sturdy box approximately 12 inches high. A measuring scale is placed on top of the box with the 9-inch mark even with the near edge of the box. The "zero" end of the ruler is nearest the student.

Test Description: The student removes his/her shoes and sits down at the test apparatus. One leg is fully extended with the foot flat against the end of the box. The other knee is bent with the sole of the foot flat on the floor and 2 to 3 inches to the side of the straight knee. The arms are extended forward over the measuring scale with the hands placed one on top of the other (see Figure 13). With palms down, the student reaches directly forward with both hands along the scale four times and holds the position of the fourth reach for at least 1 second (see Figure 14). After measuring one side, the student switches the

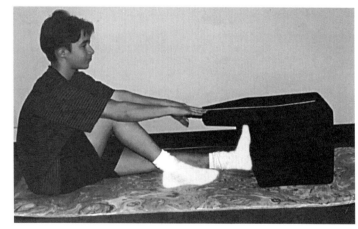

Figure 13. *Starting position.*

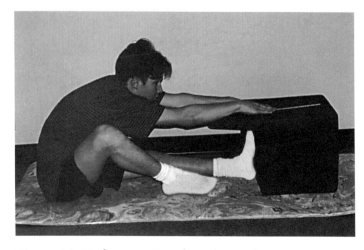

Figure 14. *Back-saver sit-and-reach stretch.*

position of the legs and reaches again. The student may allow the bent knee to move to the side as the body moves by it, if necessary.

Scoring: Record the number of inches on each side to the last whole inch reached to a maximum score of 12 inches. The Prudential FITNESSGRAM will report this score as "P" (pass) or "F" (fail) depending upon the distance reached as it compares to the appropriate standard.

Suggestions for Test Administration:

◆ It is permissible for the bent knee to move to the side, allowing the body to move past it.
◆ The knee of the extended leg should remain straight. Tester may place one hand on the student's knee to remind him/her to keep the knee straight.
◆ Hands should reach forward evenly.
◆ The trial should be repeated if the hands reach unevenly or the knee bends.
◆ Hips must remain square to the box. Do not allow student to turn hip away from the box as he/she reaches.

Shoulder Stretch

The shoulder stretch is a simple test of upper body flexibility. If used alternately with the back-saver sit-and-reach, it may be useful in educating students that flexibility is important in all areas of the body, not just the hamstring muscles.

Test Objective: To be able to touch the fingertips together behind the back by reaching over the shoulder and under the elbow.

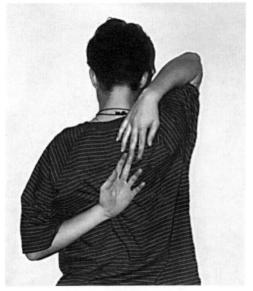
Figure 15. Shoulder stretch on right side.

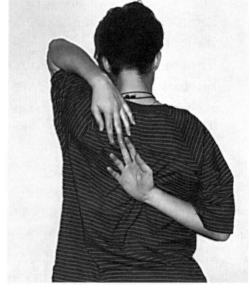
Figure 16. Shoulder stretch on the left side.

Equipment/Facilities: No equipment is necessary to complete this test item.

Test Description: Allow students to select a partner. Partner judges ability to complete the stretch.

To test right shoulder, the student reaches with right hand over right shoulder and down the back as if to pull up a zipper. At the same time, the student places the left hand behind back and reaches up trying to touch the fingers of the right hand (see Figure 15). Partner observes if fingers touch.

To test left shoulder, student reaches with left hand over left shoulder and down the back as if to pull up a zipper. At the same time, the student places the right hand behind back and reaches up trying to touch the fingers of the left hand (see Figure 16).

Scoring: The test is scored pass/fail. If the student is able to touch the fingers with right hand over the shoulder, a "P" is recorded for the right side, or else an "F" is recorded. If the student is able to touch the fingers with left hand over the shoulder, a "P" is recorded for the left side, or else an "F" is recorded.

Teaching Students How to Take The Prudential FITNESSGRAM Tests

Use VA 2.13 to help explain how to take The Prudential FITNESSGRAM tests. In addition to being explained, each test should be demonstrated, and every student should practice each test item. The trial performance should be on a different day from the actual assessment. You may want to try different tests on different days. Teaching points and activities are described below.

One Mile Run/Walk and the PACER

◆ **Learn to pace**—For the mile run, if the run is too fast in the beginning, the student will tire before the end of the run and have to slow down. Since the score is the amount of time it takes to cover one mile, slowing at the end of the run may cause the time to be longer than if a steady pace had been maintained. It is important to practice learning to run at the same pace for the entire mile. Several activities for learning pace are presented below.

◆ **Learn to run properly**—Running with correct form will allow the student to run longer and faster with less fatigue. Suggestions for running properly are presented below.

◆ **Activities to maximize performance on the PACER and One Mile Run/Walk:**

1. Aerobic tests often leave students with a taste of failure and resulting negative feelings about running. Much of these feelings can be avoided if students are properly prepared prior to the test. Students must understand that performance in aerobic activities is partially controlled by genetic make-up. Self-improvement is the desired outcome rather than a comparison of scores with other students.

2. Students should have participated in aerobic activities for 2 to 6 weeks prior to testing. A common practice is to test students immediately upon their return to school in the fall, even though they may not have exercised regularly during the summer months. Asking them to participate in an aerobic test upon their return often results in a traumatic experience due to poor performance and muscle soreness. Daily aerobic activities practiced before testing should last approximately 10 to 15 minutes.

3. Develop a testing procedure for the run that does not force all students to start and finish at the same point. Starting all runners simultaneously at a common point dramatically illustrates to the class who the slowest and fastest runners are. Many students will not continue to give their best effort in the run if they fall behind in the early stages of the test. Another idea is to allow students to group themselves with students of similar ability. This type of grouping may result in a better performance since students who are comfortable with each other are less reactive and critical.

4. Teach students how to pace their running performance. Most elementary school students will run as fast as possible at the beginning of the race and then fatigue quickly. They become discouraged and choose not to try. An optimum score will more likely be earned when students are able to run at a consistent and steady rate. A technique for teaching students how to pace themselves is to place cones at similar intervals and challenge students to run from cone to cone at a specified rate. A student or the instructor can call out the time at each cone, and students can adjust their running to the desired pace.

5. Another method of teaching pace is to break down long-distance runs into smaller segments and times. This enables students to get a feel for how fast they should run the shorter distances to attain a certain cumulative time over the longer distance. The following table (also VA 2.14) shows how fast a student must run 40 yards to run a mile in a specified time.

To run a mile in:	Must run 40 yards in:
6:00 minutes	8.2 seconds
8:00 minutes	10.9 seconds
10:00 minutes	13.6 seconds
12:00 minutes	16.4 seconds

Students should practice running the 40 yards at a speed which is comfortable to them in order to judge how long it would take to run a mile. They can then try maintaining this pace for 120 yards and gradually increase the distance as they develop a proper rate of speed.

6. An enjoyable activity for learning pace is to ask students to estimate a time in which they will complete the one mile run/walk. The winner of the race is the student who is closest to his pre-estimated time. Remember that the goal of these activities is to encourage students to run. Running must provide some type of challenge and positive reinforcement if it is going to be an enjoyable activity.

7. Practice running technique. Since running is often a problem for many students, a lesson in running technique may be useful. Review the suggestions for proper running (VA 2.15). Students may work with a partner to try to improve running technique. One student runs while the other student evaluates performance points. Discuss running errors and run again. Change roles and repeat.

8. When using the PACER test, allow students a number of opportunities to learn what the optimum speed is for running the 20-meter distance. In the early stages of learning the PACER test, students sprint faster than necessary. Practice will also make them more efficient in learning to reach the line, turn around, and prepare for the next signal.

9. It is not necessary to have students run the PACER until they are totally fatigued. Many students may be able to meet the health-criterion standard because they possess an adequate level of aerobic fitness. Once the standard is reached, it should be the student's choice as to whether he or she wants to continue. Some teachers have had excellent success with placing a signal on the audiotape which announces when the criterion level has been reached for a specific age and sex.

Sit-and-Reach

To maximize performance, warm-up is especially important before the test performance. In fact, students should practice doing the sit-and-reach stretch several times just before doing the actual test. Stretch slowly and hold for 10 to 20 seconds. Remember, the back-saver sit-and-reach must be done with a separate test for each leg.

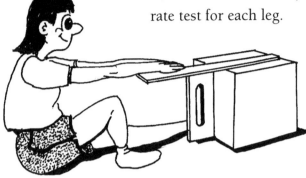 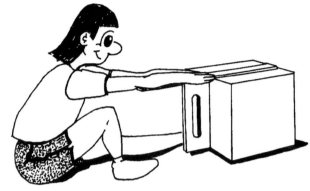

Curl-ups

◆ **Learn to pace**—The curl-up is a good exercise as well as a test. When performing the curl-up as an exercise, students should pace themselves just as they do when taking the test. If the curl-ups are done too fast, the students may get tired and have to rest. A steady speed is the best pace. Several practice trials using the test pace should be done on different days before the actual testing day.

◆ **Do the curl-up properly**—Suggestions for developing proper technique are included in the activities below.

◆ **Use a soft, but not too soft, surface**—It is best to do the test on a mat rather than on a hard floor. Doing the test on a hard floor can cause soreness to the "tailbone." Doing the test on a mattress or a bed makes the test unnecessarily difficult.

◆ **Activities to maximize curl-up performance:**

   1. Students often perform poorly in the curl-up test because they are not familiar with proper technique. If the test is going to measure maximum abdominal strength, students should know the correct method of performance prior to actual testing. If the feet lift off the floor, a curl-up is not counted.

   2. The curl-up is performed with the knees bent at 140 degrees. The placement of the heels is important since it is much more difficult to do a curl-up when the heels are lifted off the mat. Have students practice doing the curl-up while keeping the heels in contact with the ground. Staying with the cadence and learning to balance through practice will improve test performance.

3. The position of the head is important when performing a curl-up. The head is lowered to the partner's hands after each curl-up. Encourage students to "roll up" into the "curl" position. Have students try a number of curl-ups while adjusting the head position so that students realize the importance of proper head position.

4. Some students may have difficulty with passing the curl-up test. A common mistake is moving too slowly or too quickly. Students should practice doing curl-ups at the correct pace. Establishing a rhythm with a tom-tom or by clapping the hands will help teach students how fast they should perform curl-ups.

5. A successful curl-up is performed when the fingers slide from one side of the measuring strip to the other. Students should practice the movement. The best performance will occur when curl-ups are performed in a controlled manner, with the least amount of travel of the hips. It is important that the shoulders lift up so that the shoulder blades clear the floor. Some students may only move the arms, in which case the test is invalid.

Other Suggestions for Measuring Curl-up Distances

There are many ways to measure the distance traveled in the curl-up test. The important factor is to ensure that the student is moving the fingertips 3 inches for ages 5 to 9 years and 4½ inches for ages 10 to 17+. Another factor to consider is that the student should be able to "feel" the stopping point rather than relying on "seeing" it. Do not be afraid to experiment with other methods to measure this distance.

1. Use tape and a pencil to indicate the marks. Put tape on the mat at the starting point for the fingertips. Tape a pencil to the mat, parallel to the starting line, at the stopping point (3 or 4½ inches).

2. Use tape and a yardstick to indicate the marks. Put tape on the mat at the starting point for the fingertips. Have the third partner standing astride the person doing curl-ups secure a yardstick placed on the mat under the knees and parallel to the starting line. The yardstick should be placed either 3 or 4½ inches from the starting line.

3. Permanent measuring strips could be cut from a sheet of ¼ inch plywood. These would need to be carefully sanded to prevent splinters. Laminated poster board would also provide more permanent measuring strips.

4. Measuring cards could be cut the appropriate width (3 or 4½ inches) out of index cards. Two would be needed for every two students. Cards would need to be

taped to the mat in position for student to slide the fingers from one edge of the card to the other.

Note: A special curl-up measurement device is available from NOVEL Products (see chapter 7, *Sources for Equipment*).

Push-ups

◆ **Keeping the body straight**—Keeping the body straight is a problem for some students, especially younger students. It may help to practice a "knee push-up" first to give students confidence and so they can learn how it feels to have the body straight (rear not too high and back not swaying). Practice of the actual test is also useful.

◆ **Correct elbow bend**—It takes practice to learn how much bend in the elbows is correct. Have students practice with a partner providing feedback in a nontesting situation. A tap on the back of the upper arm by a partner when a 90 degree angle is reached helps students learn proper technique.

◆ **Practice correct timing**—As with the curl-up, pacing is important for the push-up test. Establishing a rhythm with a tom-tom or by clapping the hands will help teach students correct pace.

◆ **Position of the hands is important**—Have students practice correct hand placement prior to actual testing. Common errors are hands too far apart or too far forward.

Pull-up, Modified Pull-up, or Flexed-Arm Hang

Techniques for improving test performance on these upper-body strength test are listed below.

◆ **Avoid swinging or bouncing**—Many people lose their grip on the bar before their arms tire. If the body bounces or swings, it is harder to keep your grip.

◆ **Improve the grip**—A towel should be used to dry the bar if it becomes sweaty from the preceding person. The towel may also be used to dry the hands if they get sweaty before beginning the test. Chalk used by gymnasts can also be put on the bar or on the hands to keep the grip dry. Teachers should provide the chalk if possible.

◆ **Pacing is important**—Learn to pace, as for other test items.

Skinfold Measurements

Body composition measurements using skin calipers give an indication of an individual's percent of body fat. Since muscle and bone tissue is more dense than fat, it is possible to lose fat and gain weight if muscle tissue is increased. This fact makes scale weight a misleading measurement in terms of indicating changes in muscle, bone, and fat with weight reduction.

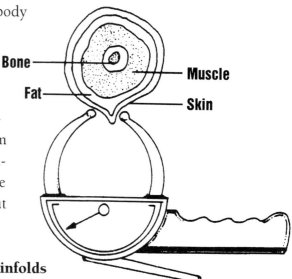

One of the most feasible methods for estimating body fat is to measure the thickness of skinfolds. A large part of the body fat is stored under the skin. Formulas have been developed which are related to the thickness of the skinfold and give an estimate of the percentage of body fat. Students should learn to measure skinfolds accurately so they will be able to use them throughout life. The two skinfold sites used in The Prudential FITNESSGRAM test are the triceps and calf. Try the activities listed here to assist students in learning about the measurement of skinfolds.

◆ **Allow students the opportunity to measure the skinfolds on a partner of their choice**—Have students add their scores together, use the skinfold conversion chart (VA 2.16a and 2.16b), and evaluate them using The Prudential FITNESSGRAM health-reference standards (VA 2.5 and 2.6).
◆ **Have students use a caliper to measure skinfolds on friends and parents.**
◆ **Discuss with students the importance of maintaining body fat within the optimal range.**
◆ **Discuss problems that could develop if a person attempts to maintain an excessively low percentage of body fat**—These problems include bulimia, anorexia, amenorrhea, and a deficiency in calcium deposition. Problems that occur when informing students about their body composition can be exaggerated due to the impact of television advertising with its emphasis on leanness.

Trunk Lift and Shoulder Stretch

The trunk lift is designed to measure the strength and flexibility of the trunk extensors. Students can be allowed time to practice lifting the trunk off the floor while in the prone position. The goal should be to lift the upper body slowly off the floor and hold the head upright. Allow a number of opportunities for students to practice holding and looking at a friend who is in the same position. They should emphasize keeping the head upright while in the "up" position. Teach students to strive for lifting the chin 6 to 12 inches off the floor. Higher than 12 inches is not better because it may place excessive stress on the spinal column. Use the cues, "lift slowly, hold, and rest."

The shoulder stretch is a pass–fail item and is used to evaluate upper body flexibility. This is an item that can be used to teach about genetic differences among students. It appears that performance on this item is relatively difficult to modify through practice. Some students will be naturally more flexible than others. Discuss with students how important it is to understand the strength and limitations of one's ability in all physical parameters. Even though a student may try to improve in this test, it may be that his or her genetic make-up may prevent it.

Explain That Fitness Test Results Will Not Be Used in Grading

The Prudential FITNESSGRAM program is designed to help students learn about exercise and fitness and to be active and fit for a lifetime. This philosophy indicates that the **process** of exercise is as important as the **product** (fitness). If people learn to do exercise and enjoy it, fitness will follow. If test results are used to grade a student's fitness, the product will be emphasized rather than regular exercise (the process). Students may get the message that fitness for now is the most important. This may lead to a lack of interest and a lack of effort for those who are low in fitness and who need exercise the most. It can also lead those who attain good scores because of early maturity or "good genes" to believe that they don't have to do regular exercise because they scored better than most people even without doing exercise.

It is important to emphasize that the information from The Prudential FITNESSGRAM is for the student. It is shared with family and teachers so they can help the student be the best he/she can be!

Precede Testing with a Warm-Up and Follow with a Cool-Down

Before the test, students should warm up. After the test they should cool down. They should also learn why the warm-up and cool-down are important and how to do them properly. VA 2.17 illustrates a program that can be used for both a warm-up and cool-down. VA 2.18 gives reasons why the warm-up and the cool-down are important.

Have students try the exercises. You can also have students create a personal warm-up and cool-down using the exercises in the Get Fit program. The warm-up and cool-down can be done to music, videotaped, and done each day with a different leader. The warm-up is done before the activity of the day and the cool-down after. The warm-up and cool-down should also be used on the day of The Prudential FITNESSGRAM testing.

Maximizing Student Performance

A majority of students may not be motivated to perform well on fitness tests. This may be a result of failure during past evaluation experiences, or it may be because they don't perceive it to be important. Teachers can help students give a better effort during testing by using some of the following activities.

Activity 1

Estimating Fitness

Many times students feel that they "are already fit," meaning that "I know I am fit, so I don't need to take the test." The following activity can be done well in advance of testing. First discuss the five different areas of health-related fitness using VA 2.2. Explain each of the tests for those areas of fitness. Next, hand out copies of VA 2.19 to students. Have students estimate their fitness by predicting their score on each test. The score predicted should be written on the sheet, and a pencil or magic marker should be used to darken the area in the fitness bar to indicate estimated fitness levels. If the student feels he or she is below the Healthy Fitness Zone, the bar should be filled below the "good" mark in the Needs Improvement area. If the student feels he or she is quite fit, the bar should be filled so that it is well into the Healthy Fitness Zone and above the "good" mark. Inform students that their predictions are for their use and will not be used in grading. Collect the predictions or ask students to save them. Tell them that they will use their predictions later.

After the test has been administered and the students have been given their Prudential FITNESSGRAM report, return the prediction sheets to the students or ask them to find their sheet. Ask students how their actual results compared with their predicted results. One possible student project is to have students write a brief paper explaining the similarities or the discrepancies in the two results.

Activity 2

Feelings About Fitness Tests

More than a few teachers have suggested that many students may not be motivated to take fitness tests. Students may skip school or bring excuses to avoid taking the tests. Completing the questionnaire provided in VA 2.20 may help change their attitude about testing, or their responses may help determine that testing methods need to be adjusted.

Make copies of VA 2.20 and have students answer the questions on the sheet. This may be done in or out of class. If done out of class, simply collect the responses (students should put their names on them). Responses may be summarized and a report given to the class. Be careful not to be critical of responses and not to make comments which seem to be associated with any particular student or group of students. If it seems appropriate, it may be helpful to ask students to recommend ways to eliminate their concerns. Making a list of possible recommendations may be useful in leading the discussion. For example, you can inform them that fitness test results will not be used in grading and are for personal use only. If the students respond to the questionnaire in class, you may want to have the class tally the anonymous responses and use them as a basis for discussion.

Activity 3

Understanding Individual Differences

If lifetime fitness is the goal, it is essential to communicate to students that self-comparison rather than comparison to others is important. The following activities illustrate that heredity, maturity, and age have much to do with fitness test results. Students should be helped to understand that tests are designed to help them plan personal programs. Improving is the key. Try these activities.

Compare a typical first grade and fifth grade score (or seventh and eleventh grade score for older students) on any test of fitness. Discuss why the scores improve dramatically as students mature. Help students understand that maturity plays a large role in fitness test performance. Focus on the differences in maturity among students who are similar in age, such as the 4- to 6-year range in skeletal age among a classroom of students who are similar in chronological age. This range of maturity dictates that students develop empathy and acceptance of all levels of performance.

Discuss how taller people have an advantage in activities such as volleyball and basketball. Most people are tolerant and understanding of others who are taller or shorter than they are. Emphasize the importance of developing similar empathy for those who possess different body compositions.

Explain the Recognition Program

If recognition is to be effective, it should be explained to those who will earn the recognition. The Prudential FITNESSGRAM recognition program is explained in detail in chapter 5. The information in that chapter should be shared with students before they take the test.

— 3 —

Administration of The Prudential FITNESSGRAM Test

The Prudential FITNESSGRAM *assessment is only a part of a comprehensive fitness program for use in schools. The overall program goal is to encourage students to follow several steps, of which taking the test is only one. These steps are outlined below.*

   ◆ *Get Ready for the Test*
   ◆ *Take the Test*
   ◆ *Report and Interpret the Results*
   ◆ *Exercise for Improvement/Maintenance*
   ◆ *Periodically Retest*

Testing Objectives

The testing information is collected and reported to the students and their parents with The Prudential FITNESSGRAM report card. The results are used to help the students plan regular exercise to gain or maintain fitness. Periodic retests can be given to assess current fitness status.

Testing can be done in many different ways depending on the specific objectives of your program. Prior to administering the assessment, consider the objectives of the testing program. Once these have been determined, use some of the ideas presented in this chapter for testing students.

Objective 1

School information— Testing provides information to the school for use in determining the fitness level of a group of students and evaluating the effectiveness of the curriculum as related to the development of physical fitness.

Objective 2

Parent information— Testing provides parents with information so they can help students improve and maintain fitness at home as well as in school.

Objective 3

Student information— Testing provides students with information so they can determine personal needs for exercise and fitness planning.

Some people argue that if the purpose of testing is to provide schools and parents with information, the testing must be precise. If those are your primary objectives, it would be wise to solicit the assistance of testing volunteers from the ranks of parents and other teachers. With proper training, volunteers can be very helpful.

Many professionals believe that an important objective of a physical fitness program is to teach students to test themselves. **If lifetime fitness is the goal, students who learn to test themselves will not only know their current fitness levels but will be developing skills to use later in life.** Learning to test oneself will be important when the student graduates from school and the teacher is no longer available to administer the test. Of course, a test such as the skinfold measurement is difficult to self-administer, but it can be done easily with a friend. If you believe that the primary purpose of your testing program is to teach students to self-test, interpret their test results, and use these interpretations for personal exercise planning, you may want to consider these test administration suggestions.

◆ **Teach all students how to do the testing**—Train students much as you would adult volunteers. Have students test themselves, work with partners, or work at stations to report testing scores.

◆ **Have students record their test results**—If this procedure is used, use VA 3.1 to make self-testing cards. Some teachers feel that students will report false data if this procedure is used. If the test results are not used for grading, cheating is less likely. If self-testing is done, you may want to indicate this in a note to parents which accompanies The Prudential FITNESSGRAM report card.

◆ **Have students help enter results in the computer**—Students may enter their results or help with data entry for entire classes. If students are helping to enter the results of other students, special care should be taken to ensure the confidentiality of the test results.

Test Administration

Some specific suggestions for actual administration of The Prudential FITNESSGRAM test battery are listed below.

1. **Help students prepare for the test.** This should be done well in advance using the steps outlined in previous sections of this book.

2. **Carefully read the test administration instructions** in The Prudential FITNESSGRAM *Test Administration Manual.*

3. **Obtain testing equipment.** Collect all testing equipment and make sure that it is in good working order. Sources of equipment and suggestions for making flexibility and strength apparatus are presented in Appendix 2 of The Prudential FITNESSGRAM *Test Administration Manual.*

4. **Prepare data collection sheets or cards.** Reproduce VA 3.1 or 3.2. If VA 3.1 is used, you may have students record their names on the cards. If VA 3.2 is used, prepare one sheet for each class of students and record students' names on the sheet prior to the testing date.

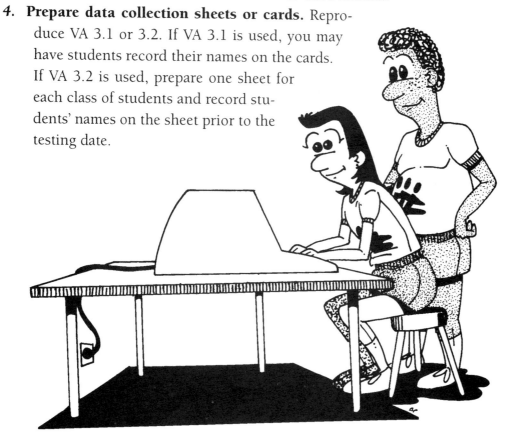

5. **Set up testing stations.** An example is shown below. Have a table or clipboard available at each station to use when recording scores.

6. **Set up testing sequence.** Divide students into groups. Assign each group to a station as testing begins. Also inform students of the sequence of testing (order of progression from station to station). Upon completion of one test, the student moves to the next testing station.

7. **Record results.** Test results are recorded at each station. If testers and recorders are used, the results are recorded by the recorder on the data sheet or card. If self-testing is done, students record their results.

8. **Supervise and trouble-shoot.** Under ideal circumstances, the teacher will not be directly involved in testing. In this manner, the teacher can check testing stations periodically to see that tests are being done properly and that results are being recorded properly. Also, the teacher can be available in case first aid is needed.

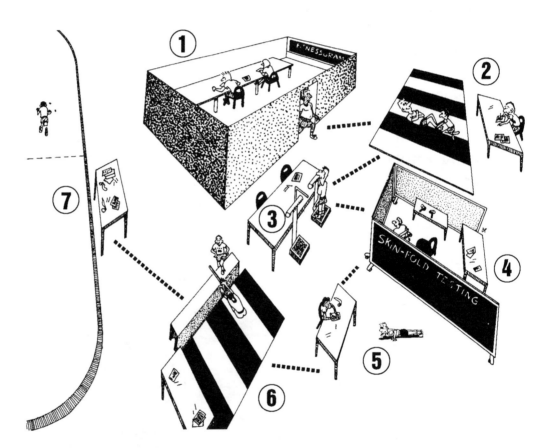

Testing Stations

1. Complete Student Information on Score Sheet

2. Curl-up

3. Height/Weight

4. Skinfold

5. Push-up (or alternate test)

6. Back-Saver Sit-and-Reach

7. One Mile Run/Walk or PACER

8. Optional Station for Trunk Lift or Shoulder Stretch

Special Considerations for Skinfold Testing

Skinfold testing is somewhat different from the other tests in the battery for several reasons. First, it is not a performance test. For all other tests, students perform a physical activity and the results are based on the level of performance (how many can be done or how fast the distance can be run). Second, skinfold tests relate to the way you look, something very important to most students. Third, it is a test on which both too high a score and too low a score are considered to be less than optimal. Finally, the test is one that is more difficult to self-administer. Special considerations must be made to account for these testing differences.

Consider These Suggestions to Prepare for Testing:

◆ **Explain the test**—Tell students that skinfolds estimate the percent of fat rather than body weight. Use VA 3.3 to explain that skinfolds measure the amount of fat under the skin. Using the triceps and calf skinfolds, it is possible to estimate how much of the total body is fat. Underwater weighing is a better but a more time-consuming and costly method.

◆ **Explain that too little as well as too much body fat may not be in the best interests of good health**—Most students know that having too much fat is a problem experienced by many Americans. Many students understand that obesity or overfatness is associated with heart disease, diabetes, and other health problems. They may not be as aware of the fact that having too little fat can also be detrimental to good health. Use VA 3.3 to point out that having too little fat can result in poor performance. Excessively low levels of body fat may cause problems of amenorrhea and a reduction in the levels of calcium deposits in bones for female students. Attempting to maintain excessively low levels of body fat can sometimes lead to the development of eating disorders, including anorexia nervosa and bulimia.

◆ **Discuss confidentiality of test results and consideration of the feelings of others**—These are important considerations for all testing, but especially for skinfold testing.

Consider These Suggestions for Testing:

◆ **Consider a private location for skinfold testing—**
A separate room or a location partitioned by room dividers will help keep test results confidential.

◆ **Partner testing**—Since students cannot do self-tests, it may be useful to have students work with partners to do the testing. You will need an adequate number of calipers for each pair of students to have one. It is recommended that class sets of inexpensive plastic calipers be purchased for this purpose. The goal is to teach students to learn how to take skinfold measurements and to assist others in taking them. Later in life a student who has learned these methods can teach a family member to take the measurements in order to continue the testing throughout life. If this procedure is used, it is important that extensive instruction be given, that much practice time be allowed, that student results be compared to more accurate testing done by the expert (you), and that students work with a partner with whom they feel comfortable. This procedure may be used as part of your regular testing or in addition to it. One major advantage of partner testing is that students who are busy measuring each other are less likely to be watching others as they are tested. This helps prevent comparisons between students. Special attention should be given to explaining the importance of using test results for self-comparison and meeting health standards rather than trying to make comparisons to others.

◆ **For the skinfold test, you may want to view an instructional video if you have not done the test before**—The videotape *Measuring Body Fat Using Skinfolds*, by Tim Lohman is recommended (see chapter 7). If you use partner testing, the video may also be used to train students.

Preparing The Prudential FITNESSGRAM Report Cards

The procedures for entering the test results in the computer are discussed in detail in the various Prudential FITNESSGRAM computer reference manuals. A separate manuals are available for MS-DOS/Windows, Macintosh, and Apple II computers. Manuals should be read carefully. Several suggestions have been made earlier in this book to help with data entry and preparing report cards. Some of these are summarized below.

◆ Set up the computer so that it is ready for data entry.
◆ Have parents or volunteers enter data.
◆ Have students enter data.
◆ Use VA 3.1 or 3.2 to make transfer of data easy.
◆ Use a Family Fitness Night to distribute The Prudential FITNESSGRAM report cards—this allows the opportunity to explain the tests and the meaning

of results to parents. Also, the recognition program associated with the fitness program can be explained.

◆ If self-testing is used, send a note with The Prudential FITNESSGRAM report card indicating that self-testing procedures were used.

Enhancing the Test Experience

The testing experience is important to the student's total perception of exercise and fitness and can have much to do with lifetime exercise habits and fitness development. Every effort should be made to make sure that the testing experience is an enjoyable one. Many of the things that make for an enjoyable experience are described earlier in this chapter, but there are other factors that can enhance a student's testing experience.

Reducing Test Anxiety

Students often worry about taking tests. In some cases, they worry so much that they get a doctor's or parent's excuse to avoid taking the test. Some suggestions that may help reduce test anxiety are listed below:

◆ **Follow pretest guidelines**—If students are familiar with the tests they are less likely to be anxious than if the tests are new to them. Assuring students that tests are for personal information, not grades, will also help.

◆ **Allow test exemptions**—If test anxiety is exceptionally great, it may be best to exempt the student from testing. Regardless of the reason the student wants to avoid the testing, forcing the student to take the test will not improve the student's feelings about exercise and fitness. Special counseling may be necessary for some students.

◆ **Maintain student confidentiality**—Since personal information about health and fitness rather than comparison of one student to another is the reason for testing, it should be explained to students that test results are for personal use. Student-to-student comparisons should be avoided. Tests such as the skinfold test should be done in a private area when possible. Special efforts should be made to assure that any student with large amounts of body fat will not be tested in front of peers. In some instances,

Most students are concerned about what peers and teachers think of them.
It is important to be careful about what you say to students in terms of their test results or the way they take the tests.

it may be better to avoid testing a student on a specific test if it causes embarrassment. It is advisable to discuss the confidentiality of test results with students prior to testing.

◆ **Consider student feelings**—Confidentiality of information and private testing can help make testing more enjoyable.

Steps can be taken to avoid hurting the feelings of any student. Consider the following:

Avoid judging student effort—Sometimes a student may not seem to be trying, especially on a test such as the one mile run/walk. If the teacher or a friend says, "You are not even trying," it can be devastating to a person who is actually giving his or her best performance.

Avoid comparisons—Telling a student that "someone else did it, and so can you" is inconsistent with the reason for testing, and it can make that student feel inadequate. Encourage without comparing.

Create a good testing environment—Let students know ahead of time when the test will be given. Do the testing on a day that is appropriate (neither too hot nor too cold), and make sure students are dressed appropriately for testing. Some teachers have "sprung" testing on students so they won't be absent. This is not a defensible educational practice.

Teach while you test—Use the testing experiences and results to help students understand exercise and fitness. Help them understand their results by discussing them.

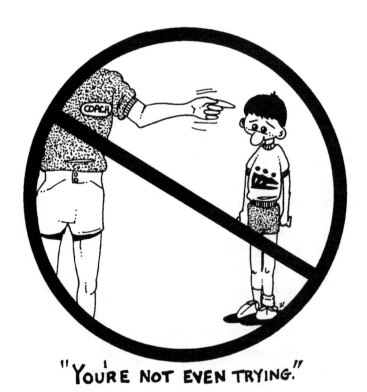

"You're not even trying."

Planning Effective Test Procedures

The preceding suggestions are designed to make the testing experience enjoyable for the student. There are some steps that can make testing more enjoyable and easier for you as a teacher. Included in these steps are the following:

◆ **Test properly**—Follow the administration procedures carefully. If you have not given the test before, try one of these suggestions:

Watch someone else test: Visit a school that has done testing before. See how they do it. If possible, watch a video of skinfold testing (see chapter 7).

Conduct a practice test: Try your testing with one class as a dress rehearsal. Have a discussion with the students during which you critique the testing procedures together.

◆ **Arrange for equipment prior to test day**—Nothing is more frustrating than trying to test without proper equipment. Be sure to arrange well ahead of time for the necessary equipment.

◆ **Record results efficiently**—One of the most difficult aspects of giving any test is record keeping. In the case of The Prudential FITNESSGRAM, not only do you have to record the scores for each student, but you also have to (a) enter the scores in the computer or (b) fill out the hand-scored Prudential FITNESSGRAMS.

◆ **Make your job easier**—There are several logistical procedures that can contribute significantly to the efficiency of your testing session.

   A record sheet: VA 3.2 can be used to help you record student test results. It is arranged to make results easy to record and enter in the computer. For the most efficient use, student names should be recorded on the sheet prior to the day of testing. Students should be called by name for testing so that you do not have to waste time locating their name on the list. In fact, you may have them line up in the order in which they appear on the list. If you have helpers giving tests, each helper should have a copy of the form and record only the scores for that one test on the sheet. The results can be combined on a single sheet at a later time. If helpers are unavailable, the tests should be given in the order listed on the sheet. This will make testing faster. The order of testing can be adjusted by changing the labels at the top of the recording sheet.

   A record card: VA 3.1 is a sample of a record card that can be used for recording test results. Use it as a master and copy it on card stock. Each student carries his or her card during testing. Students may record their results, or you may want to record the results on the card for them. Tables with pencils placed near testing stations help with student recording. If possible, each student may carry a clipboard with the card attached to make the recording of results easier.

◆ **Use testing helpers**—Parents, teachers, and even other students can help with preparation for the test day, testing, recordkeeping, and data entry.

Teacher helpers: Classroom teachers may be willing to help with fitness testing. If an excessive amount of the teacher's time is not absorbed with the testing, classroom teachers may volunteer to help on testing days once or twice a year.

Parent helpers: Parents can be excellent helpers for fitness testing. Contacts can be made through parent/teacher organizations, through Family Fitness Nights, or through newsletters sent home to parents. Simply ask parents to help with the testing. Special training sessions should be arranged if possible. Those who cannot attend training sessions can be used to record test results and to enter results in the computer.

Student helpers: Students may be useful in testing. If students are used, you may need to test them before or after school so that they do not miss the testing. Care should be taken when selecting student helpers since they will be dealing with other students' test scores, which must be kept confidential.

◆ **Use fitness-testing stations**—Fitness stations are special locations either inside or outside that have been prepared in advance for the administration of a specific test item. The location of each station is determined and equipment obtained. Student or parent helpers may help set up the stations before school. If possible, obtain an adequate number of volunteers so that each one will be administering only one test item. A table with pencils or a clipboard for each station is desirable. A possible arrangement of stations and preparations necessary for each station is presented on page 74.

Practicing the Test Items

One of the major reasons for improvement in the early stages of fitness testing is learning proper technique to assure maximum performance. In addition, this learning often improves the economy of movement and allows the student to move more efficiently. Therefore, teachers should allow students the opportunity to practice the test items prior to the actual testing situation. This will help assure that the test is measuring the actual performance of students based on the assumption that they have learned the most effective techniques for optimum performance.

1. Allow students the opportunity to discuss performance techniques. Focus the discussion on tips for curl-up, push-up, back-saver sit-and-reach, and pacing in the one mile run/walk. Students who excel might share some of the techniques which they believe help them perform well. The emphasis should be on helping others improve their performance since fitness is a cooperative venture and all participants have the opportunity to achieve recognition.

2. Allow students two or three periods to practice fitness testing with a friend. Emphasis should be placed on proper technique and scoring. Students should try to achieve their best score and practice giving an all-out effort. Just as important as learning to perform the test is knowing how to administer it correctly. Students should understand and be able to interpret correct techniques to each other.

3. Set up testing stations in the classroom or gymnasium where students can self-test on a regular basis. Make posters using VA 3.4–3.11. These posters will help students understand proper technique and remind them of important points of emphasis. Teachers using the alternate upper arm and shoulder tests and the shoulder stretch will need to create posters for these test items.

4. Give students homework that is related to fitness testing and involves the parents. For example, VA 3.12 shows a sample homework assignment which asks students to participate in aerobic activities at home.

Practicing the Test Items

One of the major reasons for improvement in the early stages of fitness testing is learning proper technique to assure maximum performance. In addition, this learning often improves the economy of movement and allows the student to move more efficiently. Therefore, teachers should allow students the opportunity to practice the test items prior to the actual testing situation. This will help assure that the test is measuring the actual performance of students based on the assumption that they have learned the most effective techniques for optimum performance.

1. Allow students the opportunity to discuss performance techniques. Focus the discussion on tips for curl-up, push-up, back-saver sit-and-reach, and pacing in the one mile run/walk. Students who excel might share some of the techniques which they believe help them perform well. The emphasis should be on helping others improve their performance since fitness is a cooperative venture and all participants have the opportunity to achieve recognition.

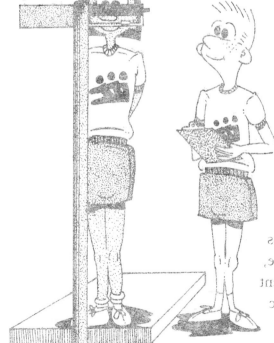

2. Allow students two or three periods to practice fitness testing with a friend. Emphasis should be placed on proper technique and scoring. Students should try to achieve their best score and practice giving an all-out effort. Just as important as learning to perform the test is knowing how to administer it correctly. Students should understand and be able to interpret correct techniques to each other.

3. Set up testing stations in the classroom or gymnasium where students can self-test on a regular basis. Make posters using VA 3.4–3.11. These posters will help students understand proper technique and remind them of important points of emphasis. Teachers using the alternate upper arm and shoulder tests and the shoulder stretch will need to create posters for these test items.

4. Give students homework that is related to fitness testing and involves the parents. For example, VA 3.12 shows a sample homework assignment which asks students to participate in aerobic activities at home.

4

After Testing: The Physical Fitness Program

Many times, fitness testing is simply an activity that teachers conduct in the fall and again in the spring. Too often, little is done between tests that will result in improvement of student fitness. The Prudential FITNESSGRAM reporting program and recognition program are designed to be only part of a total physical fitness program. To achieve success with The Prudential FITNESSGRAM it is essential that a good fitness education program, including instruction in fitness concepts and participation in fitness activities, be established. Suggestions for helping students improve fitness between fitness tests are discussed in this chapter.

Objectives of Between-Tests Programs

The most obvious reason for involving students in regular physical activity between tests is to help them be active and physically fit. However, getting them to be active now and fit now is only a part of our goal. Lifetime fitness must also be a primary concern. For this reason, additional objectives are outlined below. The Stairway to Lifetime Fitness indicates some of the important objectives of a "between-testing" fitness program. You may want to use the stairway in presentations to parent groups (VA 4.1).

Stairway to Lifetime Fitness

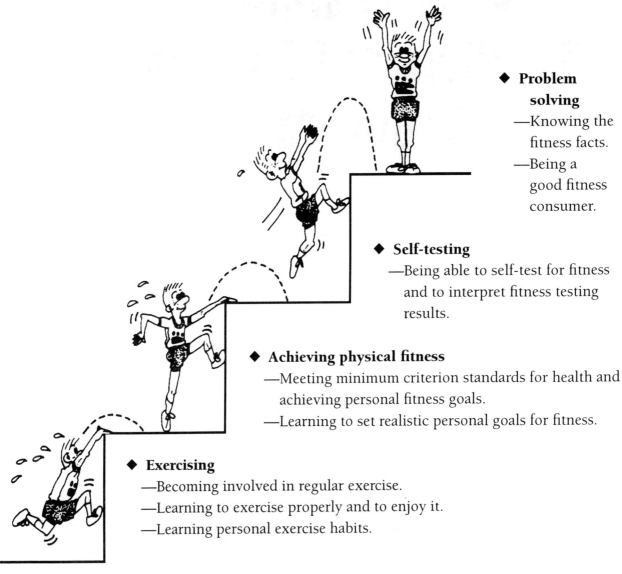

◆ **Problem solving**
—Knowing the fitness facts.
—Being a good fitness consumer.

◆ **Self-testing**
—Being able to self-test for fitness and to interpret fitness testing results.

◆ **Achieving physical fitness**
—Meeting minimum criterion standards for health and achieving personal fitness goals.
—Learning to set realistic personal goals for fitness.

◆ **Exercising**
—Becoming involved in regular exercise.
—Learning to exercise properly and to enjoy it.
—Learning personal exercise habits.

The first step in a quality physical fitness program involves students in regular exercise. However, getting students to exercise and to achieve fitness should not be the only goal. The goal is to motivate students to climb to the top of this stairway to lifetime fitness. Students must learn to exercise properly and to enjoy it. If they enjoy exercise and participate regularly, adequate physical fitness will follow. Students will have moved to the second step.

Once students begin to achieve fitness, they must learn "how much is enough." They should be taught that physical fitness is a personal thing. The first objective is to become active regularly and then to meet acceptable health fitness standards. Following the achievement of acceptable standards, it is then time to set goals for meeting personal fitness standards based on personal needs and interests. It is important that teachers assist students in establishing realistic personal fitness goals.

The third step is for students to learn to self-test and interpret the results of their fitness testing. If procedures in other chapters of this book are followed, students should make regular progress toward this goal.

Finally, students should become effective problem solvers. They must learn the skills and information to become good fitness consumers for a lifetime. In other words, a complete fitness education program includes more than fitness exercises and activities. It includes an instructional program to assist students in becoming well-informed regarding fitness matters to allow them to plan and implement their personal fitness programs in the future when the teacher is no longer available to monitor adherence and progress.

If a student leaves school without understanding why fitness is necessary and how much fitness is necessary for health, how to determine personal fitness levels, and how to mediate problem areas, the physical education program has not provided that student with an adequate fitness education.

Subsequent sections of this chapter will include suggestions in the following areas:

◆ **Involving students in regular exercise**—The activities are designed to make exercise fun. Of course, the goal of the fitness activities is also to achieve the second step on the fitness stairway, acceptable fitness levels.

◆ **Developing positive attitudes and motivating students**—Because it is essential that the first steps on the fitness stairway are enjoyable, some suggestions for developing positive attitudes and motivating students are also included.

◆ **Helping students become good fitness consumers**—Because the highest objective (the top step) is becoming a good problem solver, a good program must include information designed to provide students with necessary information. Therefore, a section in this chapter will include suggestions for teaching students the facts about exercise and fitness. Many suggestions for teaching students to do self-testing are presented in chapter 3 and therefore will not be included in this discussion. In addition, the reader is referred to the references in chapter 7, specifically the following books:

C. B. Corbin and R. Lindsey, *Fitness for Life*.

R. P. Pangrazi and P. W. Darst, *Dynamic Physical Education Curriculum and Instruction for Secondary School Students*.

R. P. Pangrazi and V. P. Dauer, *Dynamic Physical Education for Elementary School Children*.

J. B. Richmond, E. T. Pounds, and C. B. Corbin, *Health for Life*.

It should be noted that helping all students reach the top of the Stairway to Lifetime Fitness cannot be accomplished by physical educators alone. Time is limited in physical education classes. Objectives in other physical activity areas also require class time. Therefore, it may be impossible for students to get adequate activity and adequate learning experiences in typical physical education classes. For this reason, it is essential that fitness become a home and community priority as well as a school priority. Fitness activities at home should be encouraged, as should involvement in sports activities in the school and community. Physical educators must realize that they cannot accomplish exercise and fitness goals single-handedly. Assistance in reaching these goals must be solicited from parents and community agencies.

A Note About Grading

If fitness is for everyone and for a lifetime, several changes in traditional grading schemes seem necessary. As with the actual physical fitness test, it is important that performance level not be a factor in grading in the physical fitness instructional unit. Rather, it is suggested that students be graded on their self-testing skills, their ability to interpret personal test results, their personal knowledge of fitness information, and their ability to plan personal fitness programs. Since these are the objectives of a good fitness program, it seems reasonable that these accomplishments rather than performance level be the appropriate basis for grading.

Developing Positive Attitudes Toward Physical Activity

Exercise can contribute to improved physical well-being and an enhanced quality of life for individuals of all ages. Developing a positive attitude about physical activity should begin during the formative years. Initially, emphasis should be placed on enjoying activity and on achieving a better understanding of the body's capacity for physical performance. Since children are physiologically well equipped for endurance activity and therefore perform well in aerobic activities, fitness routines that promote enjoyment of vigorous exercise should be presented. The following strategies should be used to make exercise more enjoyable for students.

◆ **Instructors should individualize exercises to accommodate the various stages of physical growth and maturity demonstrated by students**—Students who are expected to participate in fitness activities but are unable to perform some exercises due to delayed physical maturity are not likely to develop a positive attitude toward physical activity.

◆ **Students should be exposed to a wide variety of physical fitness routines and exercises**—Presenting diverse fitness opportunities not only decreases the monotony of doing the same routines week after week. Diversity also increases the likelihood that each student will experience activities which are personally enjoyable. Avoiding potential boredom by systematically changing fitness activities is a significant step in helping the student perceive fitness in a positive manner.

◆ **Students should acquire a basic understanding of physical fitness**—Knowledge of the values of physical fitness, how to apply the principles of exercise, and how fitness can become a part of one's lifestyle can positively alter a student's outlook toward physical activity. Presenting planned mini-lessons about various concepts of fitness or simply calling the class together at the end of the lesson to discuss key fitness points learned during class can assist in promoting a clearer understanding of why fitness is important.

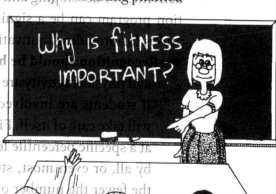

◆ **Students should be assured of success in fitness activities**—Everyone enjoys success, and students become motivated to perform when they sense that success is possible. Consideration must be given to the physical capabilities and limitations of each

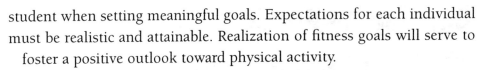

student when setting meaningful goals. Expectations for each individual must be realistic and attainable. Realization of fitness goals will serve to foster a positive outlook toward physical activity.

◆ **Teacher feedback**—Verbal/nonverbal behavior or written comments will contribute to the way a student views fitness activities. Immediate, accurate, and specific feedback regarding participation encourages continued participation. If it is provided in a positive manner, this feedback can stimulate students to extend their participation habits outside the confines of the gymnasium. In order to provide appropriate feedback, the teacher must personally believe that the first objective of the physical fitness program is to promote lifetime activity rather than the achievement of specific levels of fitness performance. Teachers must accept the premise that if a student becomes active, fitness will follow.

◆ **Role modeling**—A teacher's appearance, attitude, and actions speak loudly about his or her values and can have a strong influence on a child's attitude toward physical activity and physical fitness. Teachers who continually display physical vitality, take pride in being active, participate in fitness activities with students, and are physically fit will positively influence students to maintain an active lifestyle.

Motivating Students to Maintain Physical Fitness

Motivation is a necessary ingredient in stimulating a student to participate in activities for developing and maintaining physical fitness. The physical education program can be a significant source of this motivation. Some considerations for providing motivation follow.

◆ **Recognition should be based on process rather than product**—Exercise and physical activity are process goals, whereas fitness is product-oriented. If students are involved in the process of activity, the product (fitness) will take care of itself. Fitness recognition given according to performance at a specific percentile level is product-oriented and will not be attainable by all, or even most, students. The higher the required percentile level, the fewer the number of students who can achieve the standard. Historically, to receive the most familiar national fitness award (Presidential Fitness Award) a student was required to score at or above the 85th percentile on six test items. Results of the National School Population Fitness survey indicated the only 0.1 percent of the boys and 0.3 percent of the girls could attain this standard on the Youth Fitness Test (see Footnote 1.).

When only a small number of students are able to achieve the award perceived as most important, it may become very prestigious for those few receiving the award but generally becomes very discouraging to the vast majority who are unable to achieve the standard and perceive it as impossible. The Prudential FITNESSGRAM program is process-oriented, and recognition can be acquired by participation in regular activity.

◆ **Goals should be challenging, yet attainable**—If most students can achieve their goals through adequate effort, the goals will be challenging and motivating. On the other hand, if students find goals to be impossible to achieve, the system will become discouraging and threatening. Develop a goal chart that encourages gradual progress toward the health fitness standards through short-term intermediate goals. Once students have achieved the health fitness standards, individual goals for higher level fitness activities based on personal interests should be established. For example, students can be encouraged to participate in bicycle hikes, runs of increasing distances, community-sponsored fitness events, or sporting activities. Once again, the primary goal should be participation in the events and not the level of performance.

◆ **Bulletin boards in the gymnasium and classrooms can be used to publicize items of interest about physical fitness**—Bulletin board materials should not be allowed to become out-of-date. When an item becomes dated, replace it with new information.

◆ **Audiovisual materials should be used to heighten interest in fitness**—An example of audiovisual material that is available is *Dynamic Physical Education for Elementary School Students* (specific information can be found in chapter 7).

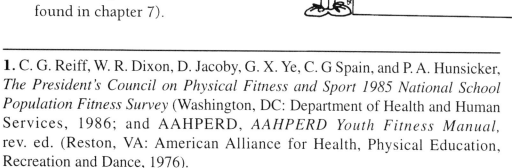

---

1. C. G. Reiff, W. R. Dixon, D. Jacoby, G. X. Ye, C. G Spain, and P. A. Hunsicker, *The President's Council on Physical Fitness and Sport 1985 National School Population Fitness Survey* (Washington, DC: Department of Health and Human Services, 1986; and AAHPERD, *AAHPERD Youth Fitness Manual*, rev. ed. (Reston, VA: American Alliance for Health, Physical Education, Recreation and Dance, 1976).

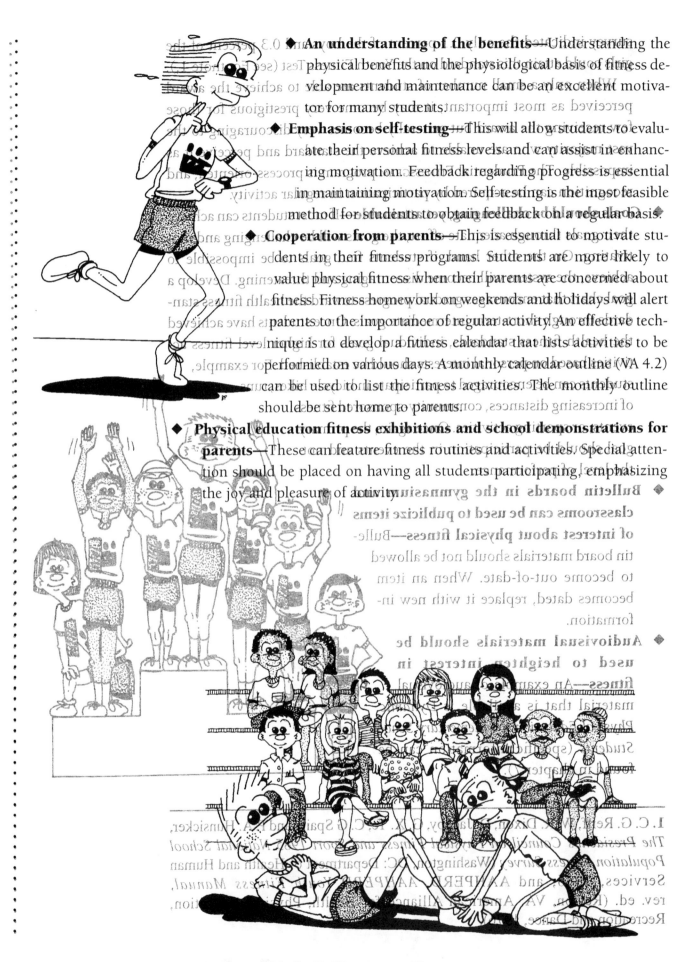

• **An understanding of the benefits**—Understanding the physical benefits and the physiological basis of fitness development and maintenance can be an excellent motivator for many students.

• **Emphasis on self-testing**—This will allow students to evaluate their personal fitness levels and can assist in enhancing motivation. Feedback regarding progress is essential in maintaining motivation. Self-testing is the most feasible method for students to obtain feedback on a regular basis.

• **Cooperation from parents**—This is essential to motivate students in their fitness programs. Students are more likely to value physical fitness when their parents are concerned about fitness. Fitness homework on weekends and holidays will alert parents to the importance of regular activity. An effective technique is to develop a fitness calendar that lists activities to be performed on various days. A monthly calendar outline (VA 4.2) can be used to list the fitness activities. The monthly outline should be sent home to parents.

• **Physical education fitness exhibitions and school demonstrations for parents**—These can feature fitness routines and activities. Special attention should be placed on having all students participating, emphasizing the joy and pleasure of activity.

Fitness Activities for Primary Grade Students

Fitness activities for young students should have the potential to develop components of physical fitness and exercise the various body parts. The entire lesson for any specific day should combine to provide broad coverage by including four general areas of the body and the five areas of health-related physical fitness.

Body Parts	Fitness Components
Trunk	Aerobic Capacity
Abdomen	Body Composition
Arm and Shoulder Girdle	Muscular Strength
Legs	Muscular Endurance
	Flexibility

Movement Challenges

Many selected movement challenges can be used to develop fitness routines for students at this level. Alternate nonlocomotor activities with locomotor activities. When students are pushed too hard aerobically, they will express their fatigue in many different ways (complaining, quitting, misbehaving, or sitting out). Effective instructors are keenly aware of how far to push and when to ease up. Instruction must be sensitive to the capacities of young students.

The approach to movement challenges should be very relaxed and informal, using directives such as "Can you...?" or "Show me how you can...." In movement challenges, students are allowed to respond individually as they choose. Remember! There are no right or wrong answers to movement challenges. If the response is not as expected, perhaps the challenge should be reworded or clarified.

The majority of the fitness activities in this chapter have been adapted from R. P. Pangrazi and V. P. Dauer (1993), *Dynamic Physical Education for Elementary School Children*, 11th ed. (Boston: Allyn and Bacon, 1993).

Activities for Trunk Development

Strength, Endurance, and Flexibility

Movements that include bending, stretching, swaying, twisting, reaching, and forming shapes are important inclusions in trunk development activities. No particular continuity exists, except that activities should move from simple to more complex. A logical approach is to select one or more movements and to use them as the theme for the day. Vary the starting position using standing, lying, kneeling, or sitting. From the selected position, challenge the student to perform varied movements based on the theme for the day. Examples of a variety of trunk movements follow.

◆ **Bending—**

Bend in different ways.

Bend as many parts of the body as you can.

Make different shapes by bending two, three, and four parts of the body.

Bend the arms and knees in different ways and on different levels.

Try different ways of bending the fingers and wrist of one hand against the other. Use some resistance. (Explain resistance.) Add body bends.

◆ **Stretching—**

Keeping one foot in place, stretch your arms in different directions, stepping as you move with the free foot. Stretch at different levels.

Lying on the floor, stretch one leg different ways in space. Stretch one leg in one direction and the other in another direction.

Stretch as slowly as you wish and then snap back to original position.

Stretch with different arm–leg combinations in several directions.

See how much space on the floor you can cover by stretching. Show us how big your space is.

Combine bending and stretching movements.

◆ **Swaying and twisting—**

Sway your body back and forth in different directions. Change the position of your arms.

Sway your body while bending over.

Select a part of the body and twist it as far as you can in one direction and then in the opposite direction.

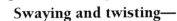

Twist your body at different levels.

Twist two or more body parts at the same time.

Twist one part of your body while untwisting another.

Twist your head as far back as you can.

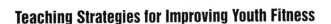

Twist like a spring. Like a screwdriver.

Stand on one foot and twist your body. Untwist.

From a seated position, make different shapes by twisting.

◆ **Forming shapes—**

Students like to form shapes with their bodies, and this interest should be used in trunk development activities. Shapes can be formed in almost any position (standing, lying, sitting), while balancing on parts of the body, or while moving. Shapes can be curled or stretched, narrow or wide, big or little, symmetrical or asymmetrical, twisted or straight.

Activities for the Development of the Abdominal Region

Strength and Endurance

The best position for exercising the abdominal muscles is supine on the floor or on a mat. In general, the legs should be lifted one at a time. If lifting both legs, bring the knees to the chest and then extend the legs. To lower, reverse this movement.

The following are possible directives.

—Sit up and touch both knees with your elbows (arms across chest).

—Sit up and touch your right knee with your left elbow. Do it the other way.

—With hands to the side, bring your knees to the chest and then straighten your legs up into the air. Touch your feet with the right hand and then with the left hand. Do not lift straight legs simultaneously.

—Lift your head from the floor and look at your toes. Wink your right eye and wiggle your left foot. Reverse.

—Bring your knees to your chest. Touch your left knee with your right elbow. Reverse. Touch both knees with elbows.

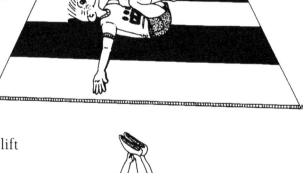

Activities for the Development of the Arm and Shoulder Girdle

Strength

For young students, movement challenges done from a push-up position can be fun and provide beginning-level strength development activities for the upper body. With slight modifications, the challenges can also be issued from the crab position or a side-leaning position. Strength development results from maintaining the support of the body on the arms for a period of time.

Each student assumes the push-up position, which provides a base of operation. The challenges require a movement and then a return to the original position. If the challenges are too difficult, they can be performed with one knee on the floor.

—Lift one foot high. Now the other foot.

—Bounce both feet up and down. Move the feet out from each other while bouncing.

—Inch the feet up to the hands and go back again. Inch the feet up to the hands, and then inch the hands out to return to the original position.

—Reach up with one hand and touch the other shoulder behind the back.

—Lift both hands from the floor. Try clapping the hands.

—Bounce from the floor with both hands and feet off the floor at the same time.

—Turn over so that the back is to the floor. Now complete the turn to the original position.

—Lower the body an inch at a time until the chest touches the floor. Return.

Activities for the Development of the Legs

Strength, Aerobic Capacity, Body Composition

Activities to develop leg strength can include a wide range of movement challenges, either in general space or in place. In general, activities that develop leg strength will also help in the development of aerobic capacity. The introductory phase of the lesson often incorporates some type of running activity. Most of the activities in this section work best when interspersed with trunk, abdominal, and arm–shoulder girdle development activities.

◆ **Running Patterns—**

Running in place: Alternate between slow and fast running. Use the words "tortoise" and "hare" to signal slow and fast paces.

Home and away: Students use a carpet square, bean-bag, or hoop to designate their home space. On signal they move away from home. On the second signal, they quickly return home.

Running and stopping: Practice moving "like an athlete." This means moving the body under control. Too often students move out of control, resulting in collisions. Athletes seldom "crash" because they have learned to manage their bodies well.

Running and changing direction on signal: This activity is excellent for teaching students to move and respond to a signal. The goal is to move under control, yet change direction quickly. Use the PACER tape and have students change direction or freeze on each signal.

◆ **Jumping and hopping patterns—**

Jump or hop in different directions back and forth over a spot on the floor.

Jump or hop in, out, over, and around hoops, individual mats, or jump ropes laid on the floor.

Individual rope jumping: Allow students the choice as to what type of jumping skill they use.

◆ **Locomotor movement combinations—**

Many combinations of locomotor movements can be suggested. Examples are run, leap, and roll; or run, jump-turn, and skip. The number of possible combinations is limited only by the imagination of the teacher and the students.

Sample Routines

Combinations of Abdominal Development Activities

—In a sitting position, who can pick up one leg and shake it? Now the other. (Do not lift both legs at once).

—In a sitting position with knees bent, who can lean the upper body backward without falling? How long can you hold this position?

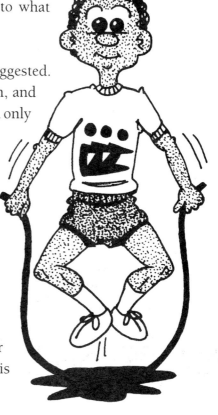

—From a sitting position, who can lower themselves slowly to the floor? Now, can you sit up?

—In a supine position, who can lift their head and look at their toes? Can you see your heels? Who can see the back of their knees?

—In a supine position, who can "wave" a leg at a friend? Use the other leg. (Do not lift both legs at the same time.)

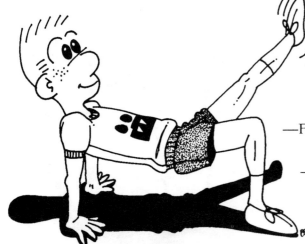

—From a supine position with knees bent, who can sit up and touch their toes?

—From a supine position, who can hold their shoulders off the floor?

—From a sitting position, who can lift their legs off the floor and at the same time touch their toes with their fingers?

—From a supine position with knees bent, who can sit up with hands placed on tummy? With hands folded across the chest? With hands placed on top of head?

Combinations of Arm–Shoulder Girdle Development Activities

—Can you walk on your hands and feet?

—Can you walk on two hands and one foot?

—Can you walk on one hand and one foot?

—Can you walk in the crab position (tummy toward the ceiling)?

—In crab position, can you wave an arm at a friend? Can you wave a foot at a friend?

—How long can you hold a bridge position (push-up position)?

—Who can walk to this line in the push-up position?

—Who can scratch their back with the right hand while maintaining the push-up position? With the left hand?

—Can anyone clap their hands while holding the push-up position?

—Starting in the push-up position, walk the feet to the hands and back to the original position. Who can walk just one foot forward?

—From the push-up position, lower the body 1 inch at a time. Can you move 5 inches?

—From the push-up position, turn over and face the ceiling.

Combinations of Leg Development Activities

—Who can run in place? Who can do 50 running steps in place without stopping?
—Who can do 40 skips or gallops?
—Who can slide all the way around the gymnasium?
—Who can hop 30 times on the left foot?
—Who can jump in place 40 times?
—Who can jump in place while twisting the arms and upper body?
—Who can do 10 skips, 10 gallops, and finish with 30 running steps?
—Who can hold hands with a partner and run 20 steps and do 50 jumps?
—Who can skip or gallop to the other side of the gymnasium carrying a jump rope and then jump the rope 50 times?
—Who can hop back and forth over this line for 20 hops and then jump over the line 20 jumps?
—Try to run as fast as you can. How long can you keep going?

Combination Movement Challenges

The objective in activities that combine movement challenges should be to combine different types of locomotor movements with nonlocomotor movements. Locomotor movements include walking, running, skipping, galloping, hopping, jumping, leaping, and sliding. Nonlocomotor movements might include twisting, turning, rolling, rocking, bending, swinging, stretching, pushing, and pulling. Overload and progression can be developed by increasing the amount of time devoted to the locomotor movements and reducing the amount of nonlocomotor movement. Movements can be stimulated by following the leader, announcing the sequence, or encouraging students to develop their own sequences. The following examples are combinations that would be appropriate for a fitness module.

Sample Routines

—Run, freeze, and stretch.
—Skip, jump in place, and twist in four different ways.
—Perform 30 slide steps, change direction every 5 slides.
—Gallop, find a partner and pull, stretch with a partner.
—Try to do 35 skips, 20 hops, stop and do three different types of rocking movements.

—Balance on one body part, swing with a partner, run sideways throughout the area.
—Run, leap, roll, and rock. Repeat the sequence five times.
—Develop a sequence that includes walking, moving backwards, changing directions, stretching, and twisting. How many different sequences can you think of using these movements?

Animal Movements

Animal movements are excellent activities for developing fitness because they develop both aerobic capacity and strength. They are particularly enjoyable for primary grade students because they can mimic the sounds and movements of the animals. Most of the animal movements are done with the body weight on all four limbs. This assures that the upper body receives activity to stimulate the development of muscular strength. Students can be challenged to move randomly throughout the area, across the gymnasium, or between cones delineating a specific distance. The distanced moved can be lengthened, or the amount of time each walk is performed can be increased to assure that overload occurs. The following are examples of animal walks that can be used. Many more can be created by simply asking the students to see if they can move like a specific animal.

—*Puppy walk:* Move on all fours (not the knees). Keep the head up and move lightly.
—*Lion walk:* Move on all fours while keeping the back arched. Move deliberately and lift the "paws" to simulate moving without a sound.
—*Elephant walk:* Move heavily throughout the area, swinging the head back and forth like the elephant's trunk.
—*Seal walk:* Move using the arms to propel the body. The legs are allowed to drag along the floor much as a seal would move.

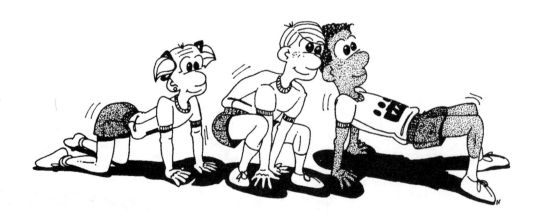

—*Injured coyote:* Move using only three limbs. Hold the injured limb off the floor. Vary the walk by specifying which limb is injured.

—*Crab walk:* Move on all fours with the tummy facing the ceiling. Try to keep the back as straight as possible.

—*Rabbit walk:* Start in a squatting position with hands on the floor. Reach forward with the hands and support the body weight. Jump both feet toward the hands. Repeat the sequence.

Fitness Games

Fitness games are excellent for developing aerobic capacity and creating a high degree of motivation. **The emphasis for fitness games should be that all students are moving all of the time.** One of the best ways to assure continuous movement for all participants is to play games that do not involve elimination of the players. Games of tag are exceptional fitness activities. To ensure continuous movement, the player who tags is no longer "it" and the person tagged becomes "it." Constant changing of the "it" makes it difficult for players to tell who is actually "it," which is desirable since it assures that players cannot stop and stand when the "it" player is a significant distance from them. If various games stipulate a "safe" position, allow the player to remain in this position for a maximum of 5 seconds. This will assure that activity continues. The following are examples of games that can be played.

—*Stoop tag:* Players cannot be tagged when they stoop.

—*Back-to-back tag:* Players are safe when they stand back-to-back with another person. Other positions can be designated, such as toe-to-toe, knee-to-knee, knee-to-elbow, and so on.

—*Train tag:* Form groups of three or four, and make a train by holding the hips of the other players. Three or four players designated as "it" try to hook onto the rear of a train. If an "it" is successful, the player at the front of the train becomes a new "it."

—*Color tag:* Players are safe when they stand on a specified color. The "safe" color may be changed by the leader at any time.

—*Elbow-swing tag:* Players cannot be tagged as long as they are performing an elbow swing with another player.

—*Balance tag:* Players are safe when they are balancing on one body part.

—*Push-up tag:* Players are safe when they are in push-up position. Other exercise positions, such as bent-knee sit-up, V-up, and crab position can be used.

—*Group tag:* The only time players are safe is when they are in a group (the number in the group is stipulated by the leader) holding hands. For example, the number might be "4," which means that students must be holding hands in groups of 4 to be safe.

—*Hanging tag:* Players must be in a hanging position (feet off the floor) to be safe. Climbing ropes, chin-up bars, and other apparatus can be used by students to assume a hanging position.

Miniature Challenge Courses

A miniature challenge course can be set up indoors or outdoors. The distance between the start and finish lines depends upon the type of activity. To begin, a distance of about 30 feet is suggested, but this can be adjusted. Cones can mark the course boundaries. The course should be wide enough for two students at a time to move down it.

Each student performs the stipulated locomotor movement from the start to the finish line while moving from one obstacle to the next, then turns and jogs back to the start. The movement is continuous. Directions should be given in advance so that no delay occurs. The number of students on each course should be limited to normal squad size or fewer. Suggestions for movements include the following activities.

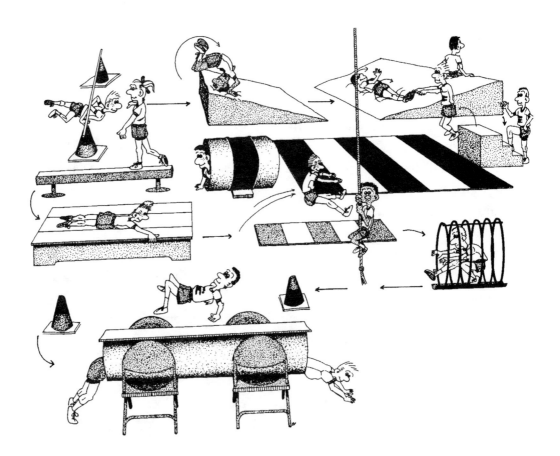

♦ **All types of locomotor activities**—running, jumping, hopping, sliding, galloping, and so on.

♦ **Movements on the floor**—crawling, bear walk, seal crawl, and the like.

♦ **Movements over and under obstacles or through tires or hoops.**

Sample Routine

Station #

1	Crawl under a wand set on two cones.
2	Roll down an inclined mat.
3	Log-roll up an inclined mat.
4	Move up and down a three-step structure a specified number of times. On the final climb, jump off and roll before moving on to the next obstacle.
5	Crawl through a barrel or one or more tires.
6	Walk a balance beam.
7	Pull the body down a bench in prone position.
8	Leap over five carpet squares.
9	Move through six hoops held together in position with carpet squares.
10	Hang on to a climbing rope for 10 seconds.
11	Crab walk from one cone to another and back.
12	Go through a tunnel formed by a tumbling mat set on four chairs.

Fitness Activities for Intermediate-Grade Students

Fitness activities become more structured as students move into the upper grades in elementary school. Emphasis on form becomes more important. When developing routines, students should be asked to perform most activities for a desired amount of time rather than a specified number of repetitions. For example, ask students to perform push-ups for 20 seconds rather than requiring them to perform 7 repetitions. This allows each student to execute as many repetitions as they are capable of doing. It is reasonable to expect the more fit students to perform a greater number of repetitions within the stipulated time limit.

The activities included in this section are intended to provide only a sampling of the many fitness activities that can be performed with this age student. Teachers are encouraged to seek additional activities and information from the sources listed in chapter 7.

Parachute Fitness Routines

The parachute has been a popular item in elementary physical education for many years. Usually used to promote teamwork, provide maximum participation, stimulate interest, or play games, the parachute has been overlooked as a tool to develop physical fitness. By combining vigorous shaking movements, locomotor movements in a circle, and selected exercises while holding the chute, exciting fitness routines can be developed.

Sample Routine

1. Jog in a circular manner, holding the chute in the left hand.
2. Stop. Grip the chute with two hands and make small and/or big waves.
3. Slide to the right for 16 counts. Repeat to the left for 16 counts.
4. Stop. Lie on back, legs under the chute with knees flexed and feet flat on the floor. Pull the chute to the chin until it becomes taut. Perform sit-up exercise (12 to 16 repetitions) while holding the chute with both hands.
5. Hold the chute with overhand grip and skip (20 to 30 seconds).

6. Stop. Face the center of the chute, spread legs slightly, and flex knees slightly. Pull chute down toward legs. Hold for 5 to 10 seconds. Repeat 3 to 6 times.

7. Run in place while holding the chute at different levels. Continue for 20 to 30 seconds.

8. Sit with legs extended under the chute and arms extended forward holding the chute taut. Using only the muscles of the buttocks, move to the center of the chute. Return to the original position. Repeat the sequence 4 to 8 times.

9. Set the chute on the ground. Ask students to jog away from the chute (for 30 seconds) on signal (whistle or drum) and return to chute at same running pace.

10. Facing away from the chute and using an overhand grip, hold the chute above the head with arms extended and pull as hard as possible without losing balance. Hold position for 3 to 5 seconds. Repeat 4 to 6 times.

11. Jump up and down as quickly as possible while shaking the chute (15 to 20 seconds).

12. Make a dome by lifting the chute above the head and bringing it to the floor. Holding the edge of the chute down with both hands, do as many push-ups as possible before the center of the chute touches the floor.

13. Hop to the right for 8 counts, then to the left for 8 counts. Repeat 3 to 5 times.

14. Conclude by making a dome and having everyone move inside the chute and sit on the rim with back supporting the dome. Rotate trunk to the left for 10 seconds, then to the right for 10 seconds.

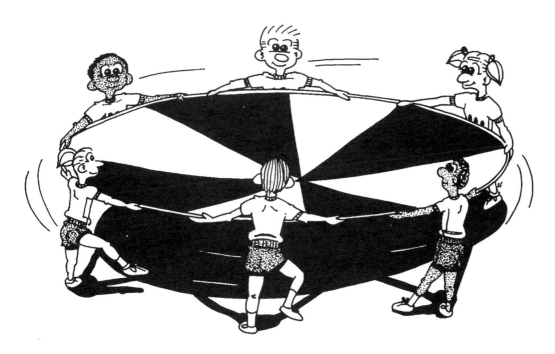

Walk, Trot, and Sprint

Four cones can outline a square or rectangular area 30 to 40 yards on a side. Indoors, the perimeter of the gymnasium is used. Students are scattered around the perimeter of the area, all facing the same direction. Signals are given with a whistle or other designated sounding device. On the first whistle, the students begin to walk. On the next whistle, they change to a trot. On the third whistle, they run as rapidly as they can. Finally, on the fourth whistle, they walk again. The cycle is repeated as many times as the capacity of the students allows. Faster-moving students should pass on the outside of the area.

Different locomotor movements such as skipping, galloping, and sliding can be used for variation. At regular intervals, students should be stopped so that they can perform various stretching or strength development exercises, allowing short rest periods between bouts of aerobic activity. Examples of exercises might be push-ups, bent-leg sit-ups, touching the toes, partner resistance activities, or any other challenge movements.

Four-Corners Movement

A rectangle is formed by four cones. The students move around the rectangle. Each time a student goes around a corner, the movement pattern is changed. On long sides, rapid movements such as running, skipping, or sliding should be designated. Moving along the short sides, the student can hop, jump, or do animal walks. Vary clockwise and counterclockwise directions.

Using the four-corners idea as a basis, other combinations can be devised. For example, students could be required to run along one long side and slide along the other. The short sides could require an animal walk on one and three forward rolls on the other (tumbling mats would be placed on the short side for the forward rolls).

The size of the rectangle may vary according to the ages of the students and the movement tasks used. Outdoors, four rectangles can be set up. Indoors, at least two rectangles should be established. Too much crowding and interference occur when only one rectangle is used for the average-sized class.

Random-Running Program

This program is effective in developing aerobic capacity in a minimal amount of time. Using this approach, the classroom teacher sends students outside to run randomly in any direction at their own speed. Students should be encouraged to run at a pace which allows them to converse with a friend.

The selection of a friend is important and should be left to the student to assure they are with someone of similar ability. The only teacher responsibility is to clock the students for the specified time and to encourage them to keep running. The timetable below offers a good starting point for the intermediate grades. Time is given in minutes. For primary students, the time should be halved.

Week	Time
1	3
2	3.5
3	4
4	5
5	5.5
6	6
7	6.5
8	7
9	7.5
10	8
11	9
12	10

Grass Drills

Grass drills require the student to alternate from a standing position to a down position on the grass. Activities are strenuous and are performed in quick succession at top speed. Fitness improvement is gained by increasing the length of the work period. The drills are executed in place, so almost any formation is appropriate as long as there is sufficient space between performers.

Basic grass drills involve moving rapidly from one of three basic positions to another on the commands "Go," "Front," and "Back."

1. "Go" signals running in place at top speed on the toes, with knees raised high, arms pumping, and body bent forward slightly at the waist.
2. "Front" signals dropping to the ground in prone position, with hands underneath the body, ready to push off and change position. The head should be pointed toward the center of the circle or the front of the class. The feet are extended back and kept together.
3. "Back" signals lying flat on the back, with arms alongside the body and palms down. The head-to-leg direction is opposite that of the front position.

Basic grass drills can be operated in two ways. The choice occurs after the "Go" signal, which starts students running in place

1. Continuous motion: In this method, when the command "Front" to "Back" is given, the student goes immediately to the appropriate position and comes back to the running position without a second command.
2. Interrupted motion: In this method, instead of coming automatically back to the running position, the student stays in the front or back positions until a change is called.

Numerous positions and activities can be substituted in place of the front and back positions. Positions such as crab and side-leaning rest or exercises such as curl-ups or push-ups are examples.

Astronaut Drills

Students are spaced about 6 feet apart and begin by walking in a circle or along the gymnasium perimeter. A succession of locomotor movement directives is then given, interspersed with commands to walk, or the circle can be stopped and the students can perform certain movements in place. They then resume walking. The following movements and tasks can be incorporated in the routine.

1. Various locomotor movements, such as hopping, jumping, running, sliding, skipping, giant steps, and walking on the toes.
2. Movements on all fours forward, backward, or sideways. Crab position can also be used.
3. Stunt movements, such as seal walk, gorilla walk, and bunny jump.
4. Upper torso movements and exercises that can be done while walking, such as arm circles, bending right and left, and body twists.
5. Various exercises in place, always including an abdominal development activity.

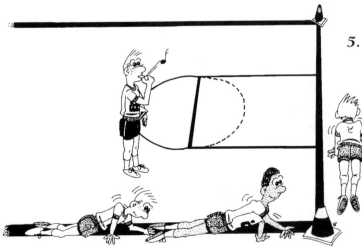

Astronaut drills can be adapted successfully to any level. Careful selection of movements is the key. Slower students should move to the inside of the circle, allowing more active students to pass on the outside.

Partner Resistance Exercises

Partner resistance exercises are useful for building strength, but they produce little increase in aerobic capacity. Consequently, they should not be used as a substitute for aerobic activities. Partner resistance exercises are especially valuable when used in conjunction with activities that demand considerable endurance, such as grass drills, jogging, or astronaut drills.

Partner resistance exercises can strengthen specific muscle groups and, therefore, have value in correcting posture and in helping the physically underdeveloped student. The exercises are simple and enjoyable; students can do them as homework. Students should be made aware of the muscle group developed by each exercise.

Partners should be somewhat matched in size and strength so that they can provide sufficient challenge for each other. The exercises are performed through the full range of motion at the joint and take 8 to 12 seconds to complete. The partner providing the resistance says "Ready" and begins the slow count while the exercising partner performs the specified movement. Positions are then reversed.

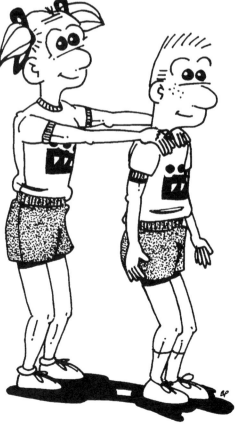

- ◆ **Arm curl-up**—Exerciser keeps the upper arms against the sides with the forearms and palms forward. Partner puts fists in exerciser's palms. Exerciser attempts to curl the forearms upward to the shoulders. To develop the opposite set of muscles, partners reverse hand positions and push down in the opposite direction, starting at shoulder level.
- ◆ **Shoulder extension**—Exerciser extends the arms and places the hands, palms down, on partner's shoulders. Exerciser attempts to push partner into the floor. Partner may slowly bend knees to allow the exerciser movement through the range of motion. Try with palms upward.
- ◆ **Fist pull-apart**—Exerciser places the fists together in front of the body at shoulder level. Exerciser attempts to pull the hands apart while partner forces them together with pressure on the elbows. As a variation, with fists apart, the exerciser tries to push hands together. Partner applies pressure by grasping the wrists and holding exerciser's fists apart.
- ◆ **Butterfly**—Exerciser starts with arms straight and at the sides. Partner, from the back, attempts to hold the arms down while exerciser lifts the straight arms to the sides. Try starting with arms above the head (partner holding) and move the arms down to the sides.

◆ **Camelback**—Exerciser is on all fours with head up. Partner pushes lightly on exerciser's back, while exerciser attempts to hump the back like a camel.

◆ **Back builder**—Exerciser spreads the legs and bends forward at the waist with head up. Partner faces exerciser and places hands on the back of exerciser's shoulders. Exerciser attempts to stand upright while partner pushes toward the floor.

◆ **Swan diver**—Exerciser lies in prone position with arms out to the sides and tries to lift the back. Partner applies pressure to the lower and upper back area.

◆ **Scissors**—Exerciser lies on one side, while partner straddles exerciser and holds upper leg down. Exerciser attempts to raise top leg. Reverse sides and lift the other leg.

◆ **Knee bender**—Exerciser lies in prone position with legs straight and arms pointing above the head on the floor. Partner places the hands on the back of exerciser's ankle. Exerciser attempts to flex the knee while partner applies pressure. Do with other leg. Try the opposite direction, starting with the knee joint at a 90 degree angle.

◆ **Bear trap**—Starting from a V-sit position on the floor, exerciser attempts to move legs together. Resistance is provided by partner who tries to keep the legs apart.

◆ **Push-up with resistance**—Exerciser is in push-up position with arms bent so that the body is about halfway between the starting position and the completed push-up position. Partner straddles or stands alongside exerciser's head and puts pressure on the shoulders by pushing down. The amount of pressure takes judgment by the partner. Too much causes the exerciser to collapse.

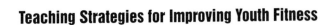

Circuit Training

In circuit training, each of several stations has a designated fitness task. The student moves from station to station, generally in a prescribed order, completing the designated fitness task at each station. The exercise tasks constituting the circuit should contribute to the development of all parts of the body. In addition, activities should contribute to the various components of physical fitness (aerobic capacity, body composition, muscle strength and endurance, and flexibility).

Instructional Procedures

1. Each station provides an exercise task that the student can learn to perform without the aid of another student. As the student moves from one station to the next, the exercises that directly follow each other should make demands on different parts of the body. In this way, the performance at any one station does not cause local fatigue that could affect the ability to perform the next task.
2. Before the students begin the course, giving them sufficient instruction in the exercises and activities included in the circuit course is important so that they can perform correctly at each station.

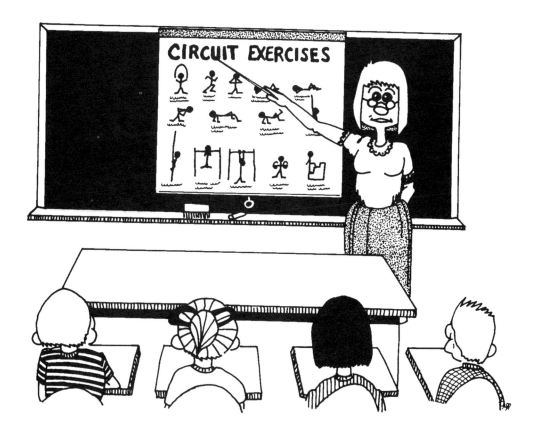

3. The class should be distributed so that some students are starting the circuit at each station. This method keeps the demands for equipment low and the level of activity high. For example, if there are 30 students, a circuit of six stations would require that 5 students begin at each station.

4. Special attention should be paid to instruction about any flexibility station included in the circuit. The general expectation in circuit performance is to do as many repetitions of the exercise as possible while at a particular station. If the exercise is a stretching activity, students should be given special instruction that the activity should be a slow, static stretch rather than a rapid ballistic stretch. Doing only one or two repetitions is appropriate.

Timing and Dosage

In general, a fixed time limit at each station seems to be the best plan for circuit training at the elementary school level. Each student attempts to complete as many repetitions as possible during the allotted time at each station with the exception of the flexibility exercises. The amount of overload can be increased by increasing the amount of time at each station. A suggested progressive timetable is provided in the following chart.

Time Period	Seconds at Each
Introduction (1st day)	15
First 2 weeks	20
Second 2 weeks	25
After 4 weeks	30

A 10-second interval should be established to allow students to move from one station to the next. Later, this time can be lowered to 5 seconds. Students may start at any station, as designated, but they must follow the established station order.

The teacher should sound a specified signal to indicate that it is time to move to the next station. A second signal should be sounded to indicate that it is time to begin the activities at the new station. These signals may be prerecorded.

Another method of timing is to sound only one signal for the change to the next station. With this procedure, the student ceases activity at one station, moves to the next station, and immediately begins the task at that station without waiting for a second signal.

Additional overload can be introduced in the circuit by modifying activities at specific stations so that they are more strenuous. For example, a station may have knee push-ups at the beginning and later be modified to regular push-ups, a more demanding exercise. More work can be added by having students run a lap around the circuit area between station changes.

The amount of activity can also be increased by dividing the class into two groups. One-half of the class is on the circuit and the other is jogging lightly around the area. On signal to change, the joggers go to the circuit and the circuit players change to jogging. Make a rule that joggers change direction (clockwise and counterclockwise) on successive runs. Try to limit the number of stations to six.

Suggested Circuit Activities

A circuit should always include activities for exercising the arm–shoulder girdle and for strengthening the abdominal muscles. A variety of activities are suggested and classified in the following section. Select one activity from each classification, or substitute class favorites that would exercise the same body areas.

1. General body activities
     Rope jumping: Use single-time speed only;
     Running in place: See page 69.
     Rubber band: See page 95.

2. Trunk and abdominal activities
     Abdominal curls: Begin in supine position with knees bent so that feet are either touching the floor or even off of the floor. Hands should be on the floor beside the body, across the chest, or behind the head. Student curls the head and shoulders off of the floor and then returns.
     Bent-leg curl-ups: Begin in supine position with knees bent so that soles of the feet are flat on the floor. Arms are on the floor with palms down. Student curls up until the shoulder blades are off the floor. Hold for 6–10 seconds and return.

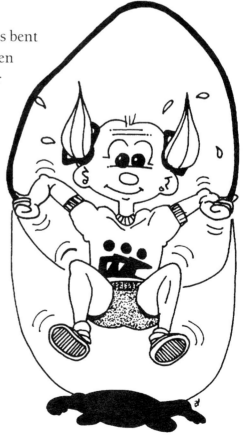

3. Arm–shoulder girdle activities
     Crab walk: Two parallel lines are drawn 6 to 8 feet apart. Start with hands on one line and feet pointing toward the other. Move back and forth between the lines in crab position, touching one line with heels and the other with the hands.

Crab kick: Start in crab position and alternate with the right and left foot kicking toward the ceiling.

Rope climbing: See page 19.

Pole climbing: See page 18.

Flexed-arm hang: See page 18.

Reverse pull-up: See page 18.

Lying arm circles: Lie prone, with arms out to the sides. Lift the head and shoulders from the ground. Alternate forward and backward arm circling, changing after five circles in each direction.

4. Leg Activities

Step-ups: One bench is needed for every three students at this station. Begin in front of the bench, step up on the bench with the left foot and then up with the right foot. Then step down in rhythm, left and then right. Be sure that the legs are fully extended and that the body is erect when on top of the bench. The next time circuit activities are used in class, have students begin by stepping up with the right and then left to ensure comparable development.

Straddle bench jumps: Straddle a bench and alternate jumping to the top of the bench and back to the floor. Since the degree of effort is dependent upon the height of the bench, benches of various heights should be considered. Benches can be constructed in the form of small, elongated boxes 4 feet long and 10 inches wide with height ranging from 8 to 10 inches. A bench 4 feet long accommodates two students at one time.

The PACER run—touch with toes: Two lines are established 15 feet apart. Move between the two lines as rapidly as possible, touching one line with the right foot and the other with the left.

The PACER run—touch with hands: Same activity as above, except touch the lines with alternate hands instead of feet.

Challenge Courses

The challenge course is becoming increasingly popular as a tool for fitness development in elementary schools. Challenge courses can be divided into two types: the outdoor (generally permanent) and the indoor (portable).

Students may run the course with the objective of completing each activity, or they may run against a time standard. A course should be designed to exercise all parts of the body through a variety of activities. By including running, vaulting, agility tasks, climbing, hanging, crawling, and other activities, the teacher can ensure that the course makes adequate demands on the student to develop physical fitness attributes. Equipment such as mats, parallel bars, horizontal ladders, high-jump standards, benches, and vaulting boxes can be used to make effective challenge courses. Variety in course design can be achieved by modifying the length of the course and/or the tasks included. Space is an important consideration in the design of an indoor course. Schools fortunate enough to have a suitable area on the school grounds can establish a permanent course. A sample indoor course including a climbing rope is illustrated below. The equipment list for this course includes the following items:

◆ Three benches (16 to 18 inches high)
◆ Three tumbling mats (4 by 8 feet)
◆ Four hoops or tires
◆ One pair of high-jump standards with crossbar
◆ One climbing rope
◆ One 36-inch vaulting box or wooden horse
◆ Five chairs

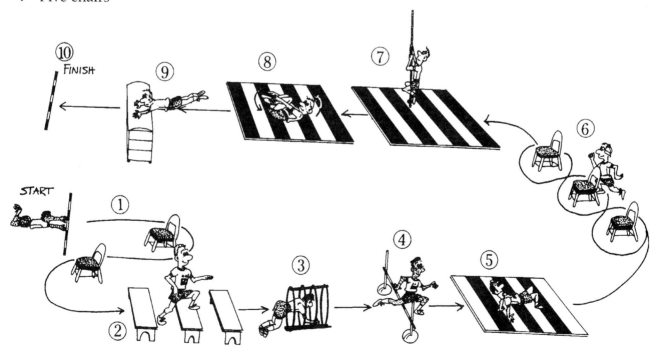

Aerobic Fitness Routines

Aerobic fitness is one of the most popular fitness activities for people of all ages. It develops aerobic capacity as well as strength and flexibility. Bright and snappy music increases effort, duration, and intensity while reducing the boredom associated with some fitness tasks.

Aerobic fitness routines include a mixture of rhythmic running, various fundamental movements, dance steps, swinging movements, and stretching challenges. Aerobic fitness movements can be high impact, involving jumping, bouncing, or high-level running activities, or low impact, concentrating on vigorous arm movements while keeping one foot in contact with the floor at all times. Music used for aerobic fitness usually has a pronounced beat and a swinging, stimulating character. Rock and roll, disco, ballroom dance, folk dance, and county swing music all serve well for developing routines. Music that is used for rope jumping routines can also be used for this purpose. Several resources that provide suggestions of specific movement patterns are included in chapter 7.

Aerobic fitness generally follows one of two patterns. The first is the leader type, in which students simply follow the actions of the leader. The second involves choreography based on a particular piece of music.

In the leader type, when the music begins, the leader performs a series of movements and the other students follow. This is an informal arrangement that depends on the leader's skill in motivating the followers and in combining movements in a manner that will ensure an adequate workout intensity for the total body. The teacher may lead, although skilled students can also do an excellent job. There are few limits to the activities that a leader can present. Those activities performed in a seated or lying position on the floor may present sight-line problems for students attempting to follow the movements. The leader may integrate manipulative equipment (balls, jump ropes, hoops, wands) with the movement activities. Movements in and out of formations are also popular with students.

The second method is the choreographed routine. For elementary school students, routines should be uncomplicated. Movement patterns should correspond closely to phrases in the music. Students enjoy choreographing their own routines to music of their choice. For most routines, music should have a tempo of 120 to 140 beats per minute.

Sport-Related Fitness Activities

Many sport drills can be modified to increase the fitness demands placed on students. An advantage of sport-related fitness activities is that many students are highly motivated by sport activities. Their enjoyment of the activity may result in a higher intensity level in their participation. Thoughtful preplanning and creative thinking can result in drills that teach sport skills as well as provide fitness benefits. The following are some examples of fitness adaptations of sports skills.

◆ **Baseball/Softball**

Base running: Set up several diamonds on a grass field. Space the students evenly around the base paths. On signal, they run to the next base, round the base, take a lead, then run to the next base. Faster runners may pass on the outside.

Lead-up games: Students waiting on deck to bat and those in the field perform selected activities (skill or fitness) while waiting for the batter to hit.

Position responsibility: Start students at various positions on the field. On command, students are free to move quickly to any other position. Upon reaching that position, the student is to display the movement most frequently performed at that position (shortstop fields ball and throws to first base). Continue until all players have moved to each position.

◆ **Basketball**

Dribbling: Each student has a basketball or playground ball. Assign one or more people to be "it." On command, everyone begins dribbling the ball and attempts to avoid being tagged by those who are "it." If tagged, that student becomes the new "it." A variation would be to begin the game by the "its" not having a ball. Their objective would be to steal a ball from classmates.

Dribbling, passing, rebounding, shooting, and defense: Using the concept of a circuit, assign selected basketball

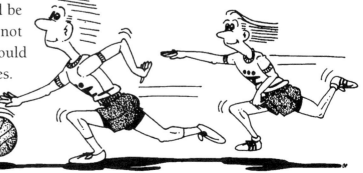

skills to be performed at each station. Be sure that there is ample equipment at each station to keep all students active. Movement from one station to another should be vigorous and may include a stop for exercise.

Game play: Divide the class into four teams. Two teams take the court and play a game of basketball. The other teams assume a position along respective sidelines and practice a series of exercises. The playing and exercising teams change positions at the conclusion of the exercise sequence.

◆ **Football**

Ball carrying: Divide the class into four to six squads. The first person in line carries the ball while zigzagging through preplaced boundary cones. The remainder of the squad performs a specific exercise. Upon completing the zigzag course, the first person hands off to the next person in line. This hand-off signifies a change in exercise for the remainder of the squad.

Punting: With partners, one student punts the ball to the other. After the receiver has the ball, the object is to exchange places seeing which student can get to his/her partner's starting position first. Repeat, with the receiver becoming the punter.

Forward passing: Divide the students into groups of no more than four. Students practice running pass patterns. Rotate the passing responsibility after every six throws.

◆ **Volleyball**

Rotating: Place students in the various court positions. Teach them the rotational sequence. As they reach a new court position, have them complete several repetitions of a specific exercise. On command, rotate to the next position. Select activities that develop specific exercise components of fitness which enhance volleyball skill development.

Serving: Divide the class evenly among available volleyball courts. Starting with an equal number of students on each side of the net, begin practicing the serve. Each student has a ball. At the conclusion of each successful serve, the student runs around the net standard to the other side of the net and retrieves a ball and serves.

Bumping and setting: Using the concept of the circuit, establish several stations to practice the bump and set. Movement from station to station should be vigorous and may contain a special stop for exercise.

◆ **Soccer**

Dribbling: Working with a partner, have one student dribble the ball around the playground with the partner following close behind. On signal, reverse roles.

Passing and trapping: Working with partners or small groups, devise routines that cause the players to move continuously (jogging, running in place, performing selected exercises while waiting to trap and pass the soccer ball).

Game play: Divide the class into teams of three or four players per team. Organize the playground area to accommodate as many soccer fields as necessary to allow all teams to play. Make the fields as large as possible.

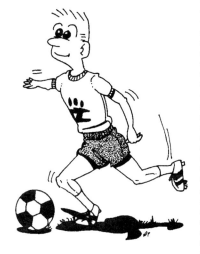

Sample Routine

By combining sport skills using the principles of frequency, intensity, and time (FIT), a wide variety of fitness routines can be developed. The following routine is an example of sport skills incorporated into an eight-station outdoor circuit.

Station #

1   *Soccer dribble:* Using only the feet, dribble the soccer ball to a predetermined point and back as many times as possible in the time provided.

2   *Basketball chest pass:* Practice the chest pass with a partner. To place additional demands on the arm muscles, increase the distance of the pass.

3   *Football lateral:* Moving up and down the field, students practice lateraling the ball to one another.

4   *Softball batting:* Each student has a bat and practices proper swing technique. Be sure to allow ample space between hitters.

5   *Continuous running long jump:* Students take turns practicing the running long jump. After successfully completing the jump, the student runs alongside the runway back to the start of the runway. As soon as the jump is completed, the next student begins running down the runway. The activity should be continuous, with station members always moving. If students are forced to

wait for access to the runway, they should be performing specific exercise activities.

6 *Soccer inbounds pass:* Practice the overhead inbounds passes with a partner. Keep the ball overhead and propel the ball forward with a flick of the wrist and proper arm motion.

7 *Field hockey passing:* Pass the field hockey ball back and forth between partners while moving up and down the station area.

8 *Fielding a softball:* Practice fielding a thrown ground ball with a partner. Make the activity more challenging by throwing the ball so that the partner has to move to field the ball.

Jogging

Jogging, a fitness activity for all ages, can lead to regular activity habits and to a personal jogging program. Jogging is defined as easy, relaxed running at a pace that a person can maintain for long distances without undue fatigue or strain. It is the first level of locomotion above walking.

The school should provide instruction in jogging techniques and in planning a personal progressive jogging program. Instruction can be offered during physical education class, but the actual activity should be done primarily during recess, at the noon hour, after school, or during other free times. Teachers may also wish to offer instruction for other school staff or parents at a Family Fitness Night.

Jogging is unique in that it takes no special equipment, can be done almost anywhere, is an individual activity, consumes relatively little time, and is not geared to a particular time of day. For most people, it is an exercise in personal discipline that can enhance the self-image and raise the confidence level.

◆ Types of jogging programs

1. *Jog-walk-jog:* The jog-walk-jog method is generally employed in introductory jogging programs. One way to apply this method is to have the student cover a selected distance by a combination of jogging and walking. The student jogs until he or she feels the need to walk and walks only until he or she feels the ability to jog again. Progression is realized by having the student gradually eliminate as much of the walking as possible while maintaining the selected distance.

The jog-walk-jog method can also be used by dividing the selected distance into specified increments of jogging and walking. An example for a quarter-mile division would be to jog 110 yards, walk 55 yards, jog 110 yards, walk 55 yards, and jog the remaining 110 yards.

2. *Continuous jogging:* The second type of jogging is to jog continuously for the set distance; the jogger increases or decreases the pace in response to the body's reaction to the exercise. More aerobic capacity is needed for this procedure than for the jog-walk-jog approach.

3. *Distance jogging:* The third type of jogging is to jog continuously for longer distances. The jogger moves at a steady pace but gradually increases the running distance.

◆ Instructional Procedures—

1. Authorities generally recommend that jogging be done on alternate days to allow for recovery from the effects of the day's workout. Some joggers, however, like to run every day, alternating between heavy and light workouts.

2. The teacher should not be concerned about foot action since the student generally uses a pattern that is naturally the most comfortable. Arm movement should be easy and natural, with elbows bent. The head and upper body should be held up and back. The eyes look ahead. The general body position in jogging should be erect but relaxed. Jogging on the toes should be avoided (VA 2.15).

3. Beginning distances for elementary school students should offer challenge, but not to the point of causing distress or undue fatigue. A suggested beginning distance is 440 yards with the stipulation that the student adjust the distance to his/her individual abilities. Students should increase the distance gradually until they are running a mile or more.

4. Jogging should not be a competitive, timed activity. Each student jogs at his or her own pace. Racing belongs in the track and field skill unit. A good technique for encouraging students to run at a comfortable pace is to have them select a partner of equal ability with whom to jog. If they cannot visit with each other while jogging, they are probably running too fast. The teacher should not give excessive praise to the first students to finish their jogging because this encourages the students to race rather than jog. Students not possessing much speed would seldom receive praise for their efforts. Another reason to avoid speed is that racing prevents students from learn-

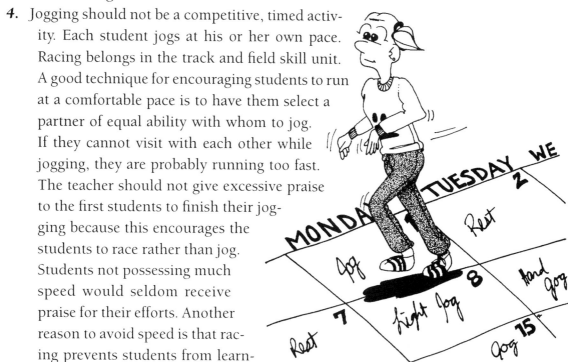

ing to pace themselves. In developing aerobic capacity, it is more important to run for a longer time at a slower speed than to run at top speed for a shorter distance.

Interval Training

Interval training is an excellent activity for young students since they recover quickly from fatigue. Interval training involves controlling the work and rest intervals of the participant. Intervals of work (large muscle movement dominated by locomotor movements) and rest (dominated by nonlocomotor activity or walking) can be measured in time. Other ways of measuring intervals is to count repetitions or distance covered. The most practical method to use with elementary school students is to time the alternating work and rest periods.

Interval training can also be done by monitoring the heart rate. The work interval is continued until the heart rate reaches the target zone, with the rest interval continuing until the heart rate returns to approximately 120 to 140 beats per minute.

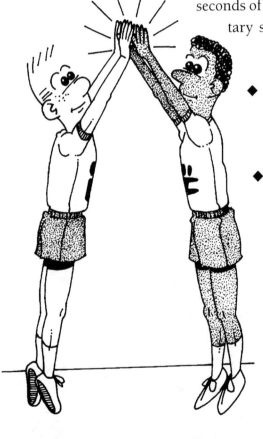

An example of interval training would be to alternate 30 seconds of jogging with 30 seconds of walking. However, to elementary school students this activity can be quite boring. The following are examples of some activities that can be alternated with rest activities.

- **High fives**—Students run around the area and, on signal, run to a partner, jump, and give a "high five." Various locomotor movements can be used as well as different styles of "high five."

- **Over and under**—Students find a partner. One partner makes a bridge on the floor while the other moves over, under, and around the bridge. This continues until a signal is given to "switch," which notifies them to change positions. This automatically assures that one student will be moving (working) while the other is resting. Try different types of bridges and movements to offer variety to the activity.

◆ **Rope jump and stretch**—Each student has a jump rope and is jumping during the work interval. On signal, the student performs a stretch using the jump rope. An example would be to fold the rope in half and hold it overhead while bending from side to side and to the toes.

◆ **Glue and stretch**—Working with a partner, one partner is "it" and tries to stick like glue to the other partner. Students should move like athletes, which means under control. The person who is not "it" tries to elude the other. Upon signal, "it" leads the other person in a stretching (resting) activity. On the next signal, the roles are reversed.

◆ **Rubber band**—Students move throughout the area. On signal, they turn and move to the center of the area. Upon reaching the center simultaneously, they jump upward and let out a loud "yea!" or similar exhortation and resume running throughout the area. The key to the activity is to synchronize the move to the center. After a number of runs, take a rest by stretching or walking.

These are only a few examples of movements and activities that can be done with interval training. A valuable addition to the activity is the use of music. An effective approach is to prepare a tape recording of popular music. For a start, tape 30 seconds of music followed by 20 seconds of silence. Continue taping alternating sections of music and silence until the total length of the tape equals the desired time for the activity. The music sequence will direct the students to perform the work interval, and the silence will signal that it is time to stretch or walk. Using the prerecorded tape allows the teacher to help students who need assistance or instruction while assuring that the intervals can be timed accurately. As the students become more fit, the length of the music bouts can be increased by making a new recording. Changing the music on a regular basis helps maintain motivation.

Fitness Activities for Secondary Students

Secondary school physical education is well suited to physical fitness units or courses. One approach is to have a physical fitness unit that includes a variety of fitness activities. A second approach is to offer units on different types of fitness activities such as weight training or aerobic dance. Several suggested activities for fitness units (using either approach) are included in the following list.

◆ **Aerobic exercise**—Jogging, cycling, walking, hiking, and swimming are but a few of the many types of aerobic activities that people select as their favorite form of exercise. Students should have the opportunity to try each of these activities and learn to perform the skills properly.

◆ **Home calisthenics**—Teach students how to do many different exercises such as those in the Get Fit program. Help them learn to combine exercises in a logical sequence and understand the benefits of each exercise.

◆ **Aerobic dance**—Have students try many different routines. Teach them basic steps and provide instruction and practice in choreography so that they can choreograph their own routines. They should also learn the difference between high- and low-impact routines.

◆ **Weight training**—Teach students many different exercises and the benefits and purpose of each. They should also learn basic principles of weight training so that they can design a personal program of weight training. Allow time for every student to plan a personal program and evaluate their work to determine if it follows effective weight training principles.

- **Circuit training**—Teach students different activities that can be used at exercise stations in a circuit. Conduct numerous circuits in class so that students learn how to organize a circuit and how to perform a circuit.

- **Interval training**—Students should learn the meaning of interval training and how it can be effectively used. Provide students with the opportunity to participate in various interval programs and to practice planning personal interval training programs.

- **Jump rope**—Rope jumping can be used as a fitness activity by itself or in combination with other activities in a calisthenic program or a circuit training program. Elementary physical education textbooks are generally an excellent source of specific jump rope skills. See reference list in chapter 7 for suggested resources.

- **Aquadynamics**—Water exercises are excellent for developing fitness. If a pool is available, students should be exposed to this form of fitness exercise.

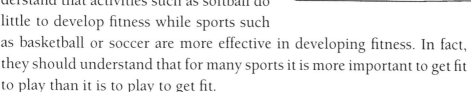

- **Sports and games**—Some sports and games are excellent for developing fitness. When doing sports and games units in physical education class, students should be made aware of the activities that can be used to develop any or several of the components of physical fitness and which activities do little to contribute to fitness development. For example, they should understand that activities such as softball do little to develop fitness while sports such as basketball or soccer are more effective in developing fitness. In fact, they should understand that for many sports it is more important to get fit to play than it is to play to get fit.

Detailed information and sample programs for each of these fitness activities are presented in the resource book *Fitness for Life*, by C. B. Corbin and R. Lindsey (see chapter 7).

Teaching Students to Be Good Exercise and Fitness Consumers

Teaching Fitness Concepts

The preceding sections of this chapter were devoted to the first two steps of the Stairway to Lifetime Fitness (see p. 58), becoming physically active on a regular basis and achieving minimally acceptable health-related fitness levels. These sections described activities that can be used to help students achieve fitness. Doing regular enjoyable exercise and getting fit for now are worthy goals. If lifetime fitness is to be achieved, physical education programs must be designed to also allow students to reach the top two steps in the fitness stairway, being able to personally assess fitness level and being a good exercise and fitness consumer. Specific content for this type of program, commonly referred to as a "Fitness for Life" or "Physical Fitness Concepts" program, can be selected from the topics in the following outline. Detailed, scientific information related to each of these topics can be obtained from several of the resources listed in chapter 7.

- ◆ **Basic principles of exercise—**
  - Overload
  - Progression
  - Specificity
- ◆ **Frequency, intensity, and time of exercise (FIT)—**
  - For each area of health-related fitness
  - For health and for performance
- ◆ **Preparing for exercise—**
  - Warm-up
  - Cool-down
  - Exercising in the heat, cold, and different environments
  - Medical readiness for exercise
  - Dressing properly for exercise
- ◆ **Aerobic capacity—**
  - What is it?
  - Why have it?
  - How do you get it?
  - Aerobic vs. anaerobic exercise
  - Facts about the cardiovascular system
  - Self-testing for aerobic capacity

- **Strength and muscular endurance—**
  - What are they?
  - Why have them?
  - Isotonic vs. isokinetic vs. isometric exercise
  - Facts about the muscular system
  - Exercise cautions
  - Self-testing for strength and muscular endurance
- **Flexibility—**
  - What is it?
  - Why have it?
  - How do you develop it?
  - Static versus ballistic stretching
  - Exercise cautions
  - Self-testing for flexibility
- **Body composition—**
  - Fatness vs. body weight
  - Effects of excessive leanness
  - Effects of excessive fatness
  - Attaining and maintaining ideal body fatness
  - Fatness and poor health
  - Combining diet and exercise for optimal benefits
  - Self-testing for fatness
- **Exercise and good health—**
  - Heart disease and risk factors
  - What are hypokinetic diseases?
  - Exercise and heart disease
  - Exercise and back pain, poor posture, and muscle injury
  - Exercise and other medical problems
- **Exercise correctly—**
  - Exercise guidelines
  - Dangerous exercises
- **Exercise quackery—**
  - Learning about exercise books and magazines
  - Learning about exercise and fitness clubs
  - Learning about exercise and fitness videos
  - Learning about exercise equipment
  - Learning about quack diets and weight-reduction products
- **Exercise programs—**
  - Learning about many different exercise programs
  - Planning a personal fitness program
- **Exercise and nutrition—**
  - Value of dietary supplements in gaining fitness

The balanced diet
Special diets
Daily food intake (keeping food logs)
Nutrition quackery

◆ **Exercise and stress—**
What is stress?
Exercise and stress reduction
Stress-reduction techniques

◆ **Attitudes about exercise—**
Why some people like it
Why some people do not like it
Self-testing your own attitude

Implementing Fitness for Life Programs in the Elementary School

Even though the content of a fitness program such as the one described above is designed to meet the top two (higher level objectives) steps on the Stairway to Lifetime Fitness (see p. 58), it does not mean that instruction in theses areas cannot begin in elementary school. It is never too soon to begin teaching the facts about fitness. Adaptation of content and teaching methods to the age and abilities of the students will be necessary. Some basic strategies for content delivery are suggested in the following information.

◆ **Mini-lessons—**As part of the regular physical education class, the teacher can have mini-lessons to teach exercise and fitness concepts at a level appropriate to the students. These can take 1 to 10 minutes and include any of the topics listed in the preceding section.

◆ **Integration with health class—**Most states require some health instruction in elementary schools. Many states also have health textbooks suited to each of the elementary grade levels. Recently, health books such as those in the Health for Life series (see chapter 7, under Richmond et al.) include chapters on exercise and fitness. Also, these books contain units on nutrition. The physical education teacher can work with the classroom teacher to teach these units.

◆ **Fitness and exercise handouts—**Many fitness and exercise handouts are available from various agencies. Groups such as the American Heart Association, the National Dairy Council, and the President's Council on Physical Fitness and Sports publish materials appropriate for use by students in elementary schools. Local health departments are usually very helpful in assisting teachers to locate free materials. These can be used in physical education classes devoted to concepts of fitness and exercise or in mini-sessions. Teachers should carefully screen free materials for inaccurate information or excessive commercialization.

Sample Elementary School Conceptual Activities

1. Have students list different types of exercises using VA 4.3. Check the category that describes what each exercise does for the body using the following categories: aerobic capacity, muscular strength and endurance, and flexibility. Determine which exercises improve all components of health-related physical fitness.

2. Ask that students exercise before or after school by themselves for 2 or 3 days. Then ask students to work with a partner and exercise before or after school for several days. Discuss the value of exercising with a friend.

3. Introduce the skeletal and muscular systems of the body. Obtain bones, charts, x-rays, and other audiovisual resources to show the various bones and muscles of the body. Discuss the effects of exercise on the growth and development of the body.

4. Use word jumbles, dot-to-dots, word searches, crossword puzzles, and other instructional games to teach vocabulary associated with exercise. VA 4.4 and 4.5 are examples of crossword puzzles for teaching fitness concepts (4.4a and 4.5a provide puzzle answers).

5. Take the class on a field trip to a local health and fitness club. Arrange for a fitness instructor to lead them through a typical workout. Introduce students to exercise bicycles, treadmills, and other equipment usually available in fitness facilities.

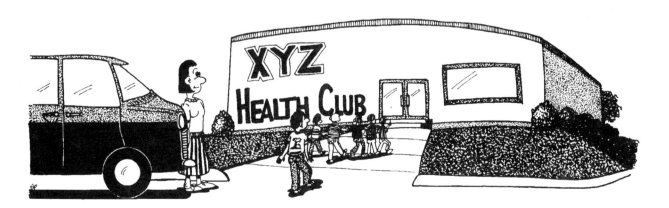

6. Ask students to list activities they enjoy. Identify the components of fitness which are developed through participation in these favorite activities. Determine which activities enhance health fitness and which improve motor skills.

7. Teach students to calculate their target heart rate. Identify activities which allow them to attain the desired heart rate.

8. Have students plan a personal exercise program. Ask them to keep a log of their daily exercise using VA 4.2. After several weeks, let them share their experiences with classmates.

9. Use various educational microcomputer systems to teach the principles and concepts of exercise. Chapter 7 contains information about sources of related software.

10. Have students measure their height and weight. Continue this on a monthly basis for the entire school year.

11. Cut out pictures of food from magazines. Select pictures which show only one food item. See if the students can sort the pictures into the basic food groups. Then make a poster of the pictures.

12. Make a breakfast suggestion box. Ask students to bring breakfast recipes from home. Use this to develop a breakfast menu.

13. Ask students to plan three meals for their family. Be sure that they include essential foods from each of the food groups. Do not forget to include drinks.

14. Introduce students to cookbooks. Let them become familiar with the terms food, calorie, carbohydrates, minerals, protein, and other nutritional terms.

15. Devise bulletin boards that show pictures of obese adults. Discuss the importance of developing a lean physique early in life early in life through appropriate exercise. Discuss the prevalence of obese students who grow into obese adults.

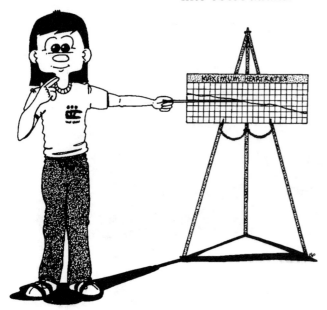

16. Conduct simulated grocery shopping experiences. Give students play money to buy groceries for one week. Analyze the purchases in terms of nutritional requirements, food group representation, and cost effectiveness.

17. Show students a jar of chicken fat. Inform them that this is how fat in their body looks. Discuss how fat is not only stored under the skin but grows around the vital organs within the body.

18. There are many educational materials which teach concepts of obesity. Workbooks, coloring books, and other media

can be used to teach students these concepts. The Fitness Finders (Feelin' Good), 133 Teft Rd. P.O. Box 507, Spring Arbor, MI 49283, is a popular clearinghouse for fitness materials.

19. Use the microcomputer to develop word searches, crossword puzzles, dot-to-dots, and assorted other games which have obesity concepts as the theme.

20. Explain the difference between body weight and percent body fat. Emphasize the importance of using percent body fat as an indicator of health.

21. Introduce students to caloric expenditure tables (VA 4.6). Ask them to see how many calories can be burned by participating in their favorite physical activity. Discuss how burning calories is related to weight control.

22. Analyze the activity levels of a hypothetical student in and out of class. Estimate caloric expenditures.

23. Ask students to keep a record of their physical activity and food eaten for 3 to 5 days. At the end of the time, have them determine the difference between energy expended and calories consumed. Class time will be required to assist students in determining the caloric value of the food consumed.

24. Discuss the ways society rewards physically fit individuals, and contrast this to the ways in which obese students are sometimes treated by teachers and classmates. Emphasize the importance of peer support to students who may be attempting to control a problem with obesity.

Implementing Fitness for Life Programs in the Secondary School

No student should graduate from high school without a basic understanding of all of the material in the outline on pages 98—100. If people are to be active later in life they must know how to be good fitness consumers. This includes being able to exercise properly, plan a personal fitness program, and choose exercise and fitness products effectively. For this reason, a special Fitness for Life program is recommended at the secondary level. Some of the activities for such classes can be conducted in the gymnasium, but others, including lectures and discussions, should be held in a suitable classroom. Textbooks and workbooks containing specific scientific background information and teaching activities are referenced in chapter 7. Several approaches are available for including Fitness for Life information in the curriculum.

◆ **Fitness for Life units**—In this approach, several Fitness for Life units are taught. The units include material from the outline on pages 98–100. The units are usually 6 to 9 weeks in length. Since all of the content cannot possibly be taught in 6 to 9 weeks, several units during the secondary school years will be necessary.

These can be placed in any of the grade levels as long as efforts are made to ensure continuity of content. Ideally the units would be included in grades 7–10 because physical education is more commonly required in these years. It is also desirable for students to learn the facts about exercise before they do extensive exercise in other physical education courses.

◆ **Fitness for Life classes**—A Fitness for Life class differs from a unit in that it lasts either one full semester or a full school year. The content is basically the same as in the units but more detailed. If a one-semester course is used, a second semester may be implemented in a different grade level.

Two approaches are commonly used with Fitness for Life classes. The **integrated approach** uses several days each week for Fitness for Life lectures and activities and other days for more typical physical education activities. In the **modular approach**, all class activities are directly related to the Fitness for Life concepts and activities. Certainly the modular approach allows much more in-depth instruction in concepts, self-testing, test interpretation, and planning personal physical fitness programs. The Prudential FITNESSGRAM assessment should be a vital part of the Fitness for Life class.

Modifying Programs and Activities for Individual Differences

The Prudential FITNESSGRAM program is based primarily on exercise behaviors rather than an attempt for students to demonstrate they are the "best." The program acknowledges and commends performance, but it places its highest priority on the development and reinforcement of health-related behaviors. Suggestions provided in this section will assist in adapting fitness activities for students with disabilities. However, the information should also be considered when planning activities to meet the individuals needs of any student.

This section is divided into two major parts. The first part deals with The Prudential FITNESSGRAM recognition program. If you feel confident in your ability to deal with students who have disabilities, reading this part will allow you to effectively use the recognition program. The second part discusses mainstreaming and modifying activities for disabled students. This part will help you develop a meaningful program of physical activity which is based on positive and successful participation.

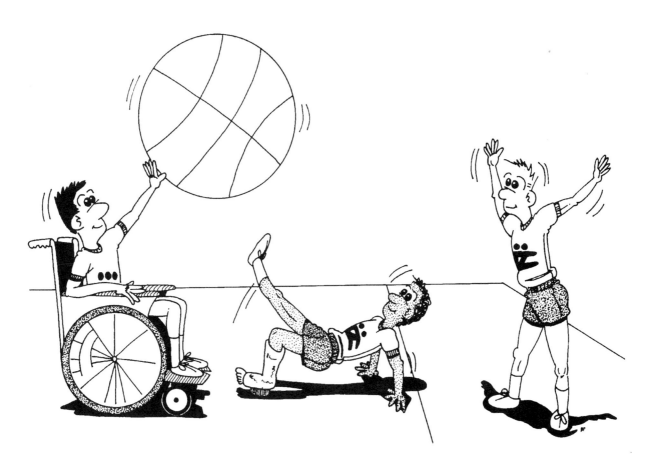

Modifying The Prudential FITNESSGRAM Recognition Program

A goal of The Prudential FITNESSGRAM program is to make recognition available to all students. Criteria for earning recognition can and should be adapted to meet student needs by using an individual contract. This makes The Prudential FITNESSGRAM program an excellent approach for motivating students with disabilities. A complete description of the various recognition programs is included in chapter 5. Some methods of adapting these programs are discussed here.

The centerpiece of The Prudential FITNESSGRAM recognition program is the "It's Your Move" program. This program, primarily for elementary school students, includes three different activity booklets with accompanying materials. Each of these booklets can be used with special populations by simply adapting activities within the booklets to conform to the abilities of an individual student. The goal of the program is to involve students in regular lifestyle physical activity. Adaptations by teachers in cooperation with parents are appropriate for using this program.

Another recognition scheme that is particularly suited for special populations is the fitness contract. The contract (see VA 5.7) must be completed by a physical education or classroom teacher with the approval of the parent or guardian and physician, if a special medical condition warrants. The contract should include information on specific activities, modification of test items, and modified test standards to be used in determining eligibility. Any student meeting the individualized criteria earns the appropriate recognition of The Prudential FITNESSGRAM.

The criteria for The Prudential FITNESSGRAM Honor recognition are set by each teacher. The certificate may be used to recognize students who have achieved specific goals. The teacher is encouraged to work with individual students to establish goals for improvement or performance on The Prudential FITNESSGRAM assessment items or specifically modified items. Individual contracts should include goals in each of the five health-related physical fitness areas.

The Get Fit recognition is earned by a student who successfully completes a 6-week conditioning program. Teachers may adjust the exercises included in the recommended program so that a disabled student has a selection of activities which can be performed in each of the required areas of the conditioning program. Any disabled student who exhibits adequate self-discipline to complete the 6-week program will qualify for the Get Fit recognition.

A student becomes eligible for the I'm Fit recognition by attaining the recommended health standard in at least four of the five health-related physical fitness components. The teacher of the disabled is encouraged to establish adjusted health standards for those disabled students for whom the recommended standards are unreasonable. It is possible that a student will be expected to meet the recommended standard for some items and aim for adjusted standards on others. If a disabled student achieves at least four of the five individualized standards, he or she is eligible for the I'm Fit recognition.

To summarize, all students are treated as important participants in The Prudential FITNESSGRAM program. In the past, disabled students have been forced to earn completely different recognition, further emphasizing their differences. The Prudential FITNESSGRAM program allows and encourages modification of goals and activities so that all students have the opportunity to be eligible for all forms of recognition.

Physical Activity and the Least Restrictive Environment

The Education for All Children Act (Public Law 94–124) uses the term "least restrictive environment" to determine placement of students with disabilities. The objective is to place each student in a setting that offers the most opportunity for educational advancement. It is inappropriate to place a student in an environment where success is impossible. On the other hand, it would be debilitating to put a student in a setting that is more restrictive than necessary. Students with disabilities, working on their own, often have been denied opportunities to interact with peers and to become a part of the social and academic classroom network.

The least restrictive environment also varies depending on the content of the instructional presentation. For example, for a student in a wheelchair, soccer or football might be very restrictive, whereas swimming would not be restrictive. Consistent and regular judgments should be made, since curriculum content and teaching styles vary and change the type of environment the student enters. The spirit of the law does not include placing the student in a particular environment or activity and forgetting that student for the remainder of the year. Evaluation and modification of environment need to be ongoing.

Physical educators most often speak in terms of mainstreaming rather than least restrictive environment. Mainstreaming involves the practice of placing students with disabilities into classes with nondisabled peers. Prudent placement in a least restrictive educational environment means that the setting must be as normal as possible while ensuring that the student can adapt and achieve success. The emphasis on placement in a setting in which the student, as an individual, can profit most is the cornerstone of the educational process.

Guidelines for Successful Mainstreaming Experiences

The concern is not whether to mainstream but how to mainstream effectively. The teacher has to teach numerous students with diverse impairments. Learning strategies with which the instructor is familiar and has used successfully may not be appropriate for students with disabilities. Attitudinal change is important since the instructor must accept the student as a full class participant and assume the responsibilities that go along with special education.

The teacher is advised to help all students understand the problems related to being disabled. A goal should be to have students understand, accept, and live comfortably with persons with disabilities. Students should recognize that all persons are functional and worthwhile individuals who have innate abilities and can make significant contributions to society. The concept of understanding and appreciating individual differences is one that merits positive development; it should concentrate on three aspects:

◆ **Recognize the similarities among all people**—These include hopes, rights, aspirations, and goals.
◆ **Understand human differences and center on the concept that all people are disabled**—For some, disabilities are of such a nature and severity that they interfere with activities of daily living.
◆ **Explore ways to deal with those who differ and stress the acceptance of all persons as worthwhile individuals**—People with disabilities deserve consideration and understanding, based on empathy, not sympathy. Offering too much assistance should be avoided.

Students with disabilities should not be permitted to use a handicap as a crutch or as an excuse for substandard work. Students should not be allowed to manipulate people into helping with tasks they are capable of doing. Coping skills need to be developed because the disabled will encounter teasing, ignorance, and rejection at varying times.

Mainstreaming should allow the student to make commendable educational progress, to understand the specific nature of his or her limitations, to observe and model appropriate behavior, and to interact socially. The following guidelines are provided as suggestions for successful integration of students with disabilities into physical education. However, it should be quickly noticed that each suggestion is applicable to teaching all students.

- In addition to participation in the regular program of activities, utilize outside resources beyond the physical eduction class, including special work and homework.
- Build ego strength; stress abilities. Eliminate established practices that unwittingly contribute to embarrassment and failure.
- Foster peer acceptance, which begins when the teacher accepts the student as a functioning, participating member of the class.
- Concentrate on the student's physical fitness needs and not on the disability. Give strong attention to fundamental skills and physical fitness qualities.
- Provide continual monitoring and assess periodically the student's target goals. Anecdotal and periodic record keeping are implicit in this guideline.
- Be constantly aware of the student's feelings and anxiety concerning his/her progress and integration. Provide positive feedback as a basic practice.
- Modify the regular program to meet the unique capacities, physical needs, and social needs of students with disabilities.
- Provide individual assistance and keep students active. Peer or paraprofessional help may be needed.

Fitness and Posture for Students with Disabilities

The mainstreaming process has directed attention to fitness and posture as factors in peer acceptance. Since many students with disabilities have low physical fitness levels, posture problems often occur in this group. One aim of mainstreaming is to make the disabled student less distinctive among peers; hence the need to help disabled students achieve acceptable posture. Values received from an attractive appearance include better acceptance by peers and more employment opportunities later in life. The psychological aspects of posture should be considered, with attention focused on the establishment of good self-concept and effective social relations. Behavior management can focus on the motivation for better posture habits in standing, walking, sitting, lifting, and general movement. Proper posture should become a habit.

Physical fitness is important for students with disabilities. Adequate physical fitness helps the student move through the school day, which may be complicated by a sensory deficit, a mobility problem, or a mental deficiency.

Care must be given to students who have been sheltered without the opportunity to participate in a physical education program. Wheelchair students need special attention given to cardiovascular development by offering activities that stimulate deep breathing. Arm development is important so that students can move in and out of the wheelchair easily.

Exercise and physical conditioning procedures can be selected to help develop antigravity musculature and to provide flexibility training. These must be combined with comprehensive movement training so that the student learns to move as skillfully and gracefully as possible. Muscular relaxation techniques may help. A well-rounded physical education program is important and should be reinforced by corrective exercises.

Modifying Participation

Special education chldren need additional consideration when participating in group activities, particularly when the activity is competitive. Much depends on the physical condition of the student and the type of impairment. Students like to win in a competitive situation, and resentment can be created if a team loss is attributed to the presence of a student with a disability. Equalization is the key. Rules can be changed for everyone so that the disabled student has a chance to contribute to group success. Students need to recognize that everyone, including the disabled and the inept, has a right to play.

Be aware of situations that might devalue the student socially. Never use the degrading method of having captains choose from a group of waiting students. Elimination games should be changed so that points are scored instead of players being eliminated (this is an important consideration for all students). Determine the most desirable involvement for students with disabilities by analyzing participants' roles in game and sport activities. Assign a role or position that will make the experience as natural or normal as possible.

Offer a variety of individual and dual activities. Disabled students need to build confidence in their skills before they will want to participate with others. Individual activities give students a greater amount of practice time without the pressure of failing in front of peers. The aim of these techniques is to make the students with disabilities less visible so that they are not set apart from able classmates. Using disabled students as umpires or scorekeepers should not be an alternative unless using student officials is a standard class practice in which all students participate. Overprotectiveness benefits no one and prevents the special student from experiencing challenge and personal accomplishment. The tendency to underestimate the abilities of students must be avoided.

Several resources provided in chapter 7 contain suggestions for modifying activities for students with varying disabilities. Elementary physical education curriculum textbooks are generally a good source of modified activities.

Physical Fitness Testing of the Disabled, by J. P. Winnick and F. X. Short, is an excellent resource for information regarding levels of performance on fitness assessments for students with disabilities.

Search for a Variety of Resources

Although chapter 4 includes numerous suggestions for activities for fitness instruction, it was not designed to provide all necessary information for teaching fitness and fitness concepts. There is a wealth of physical fitness and physical education curriculum information available. Teachers are strongly encouraged to refer to chapter 7 for a listing of resources that can be used for background information and as sources of additional and specific activities. References in chapter 7 provide a brief description of the material and give the address and sometimes the telephone number of the supplier.

_5_

Using The Prudential FITNESSGRAM Recognition Program

As noted in chapter 1, the purposes of The Prudential FITNESSGRAM program are to:

◆ stimulate intrinsic motivation toward exercise and fitness
◆ provide fitness information for students, teachers, and parents
◆ promote learning about fitness and exercise
◆ promote and increase lifetime physical activity.

The Prudential FITNESSGRAM recognition program is an integral part of the total Prudential FITNESSGRAM program and was designed with these objectives in mind.

The Recognition Program Rationale*

Before using The Prudential FITNESSGRAM recognition program, it may be useful to review the philosophy which served as its basis. The entire Prudential FITNESSGRAM program is based on the assumptions that:

◆ Fitness is for everyone.
◆ Fitness is for a lifetime.
◆ Exercise should be fun and enjoyable.

Also, The Prudential FITNESSGRAM program is dedicated to the idea that good fitness is essential to good health.

Fitness Is for Everyone

If you believe that fitness and active lifestyles can be achieved by all people, regardless of heredity, gender, skill level, maturity level, disability, or any other factor, you will realize that it is essential to **make recognition attainable by all people**. All that we can expect is that students and youth **do their best** when taking fitness tests and **do regular exercise** between tests. In fact, if all students reached their fullest fitness potential, there would be 50 percent above average and 50 percent below average. Research shows that failure makes students feel less competent. As feelings of competence decrease, students become less intrinsically motivated. In other words, if students fail fitness tests frequently, they will begin to feel physically incompetent and, in turn, begin to dislike exercise and physical activity. Thus, comparison to high fitness standards such as percentile norms can result in a loss of feelings of competence and intrinsic motivation. One need only look at the number of students who lose interest in exercise and fitness as they get older to see that traditional programs that require students meet fitness standards beyond their grasp have not been based on the notion that fitness is for everyone.

The Prudential FITNESSGRAM program is designed to make it possible for all students who participate regularly and give effort to be successful. In this way, students will feel more competent and motivated to do exercise. As a result, most students will improve in fitness.

---

*In the past, The Prudential FITNESSGRAM recognition program was referred to as an awards program. We changed the name because awards connote rewards for high-level performance. Recognition was substituted to convey the idea that all students can be recognized if they give their best effort and participate in regular physical activities.

Fitness Is for Life

One problem with fitness tests is that students are often encouraged, even forced, to do exercise to become physically fit. Programs that coerce students to do exercise may increase fitness levels for a test to be given at one point in time, but may do little to encourage lifetime fitness. For this reason, The Prudential FITNESSGRAM program is dedicated to teaching students the facts about fitness, how to self-test, how to plan personal programs of exercise, and how to find a form of exercise that is fun and enjoyable. Getting students fit for now is a worthy goal. But it is NOT the ultimate goal. If we get students fit for now but they do not learn to enjoy exercise, they will most likely not remain fit for their lifetime. The Prudential FITNESSGRAM recognition program is designed to encourage regular exercise for a lifetime. As a result, current fitness levels can improve as well as lifetime fitness.

Fun and Enjoyment

Exercise must be fun and enjoyable if people are expected to participate for a lifetime. There is evidence suggesting that exercise is not pleasant and enjoyable for those who do not feel physically competent. For this reason, The Prudential FITNESSGRAM program focuses on doing exercise rather than achieving high fitness scores. By recognizing students for regular activity, we make them successful, regardless of fitness level. It is felt that students who do regular exercise now, and like it, will be more likely to stay active later in life. People who are active will be fit. If one is active on a regular basis, fitness will follow.

Good Health Is the Key

Finally, it should be noted that good health is the basic reason for becoming and staying physically fit. Students who have fitness in the Healthy Fitness Zone not only are less susceptible to various diseases but are more likely to feel good and look their best. Beyond the Healthy Fitness Zone, each individual can choose the level of fitness that is adequate for his or her own performance or personal needs. **A premium is not placed on excessively high levels of performance on tests.** Recognition is given to those who meet the criterion-referenced health fitness standard for each area of fitness. These standards are attainable by each student.

Suggestions for Effective Use of the Recognition Program

A complete description of the various types of recognition is provided in the following sections. Also included in this chapter is additional information presenting practical suggestions to be used in implementing the program. For more details, contact the Cooper Institute for Aerobics Research or AAHPERD (for addresses and phone numbers, see chapter 7).

"It's Your Move": A Program to Recognize Regular Physical Activity

"It's Your Move" is the centerpiece of The Prudential FITNESSGRAM recognition program. This new and exciting recognition program reinforces regular lifestyle physical activity in students. Separate programs are available for grades K–2, 3–4, and 5–6.

"It's Your Move" is designed to help students do regular physical activity both at home and in the school setting. A booklet is provided that is appropriate for the child's age and grade level. The student and a responsible adult monitor regular activity and log participation in the booklet. To earn recognition the student must participate in at least 20 lifestyle activities over a period of 7 weeks. When the student has completed the "It's Your Move" activities, the booklet is returned to the school and the child's name is added to a class chart. Booklets and class charts are also available.

Students participating in "It's Your Move" must take The Prudential FITNESSGRAM test (no specific performance scores are required) and participate in activities in several different categories. Categories include: activities to do by yourself, activities with friends, activities at school, and activities in the neighborhood. A grade-related cognitive activity related to physical fitness is also required.

VA 5.1, 5.2, 5.3, and 5.4 are sample pages of "It's Your Move" booklets. These visual aids can be used to help students and parents understand the recognition program. Details of each of the three specific grade level "It's Your Move" programs are described below:

> Hip Hoppers—The "It's Your Move" Program for Grades K–2: The Hip Hoppers booklet contains age-specific activities for young students. Activities include such things as playing simple games, walking with family members, doing physically active chores at home, and doing active things at school. The student records the activities

performed in the booklet, and a responsible adult initials the activities. The cognitive fitness activities include drawing and coloring pictures of activity, etc.

Movers and Shakers—The "It's Your Move" Program for Grades 3–4: The Movers and Shakers booklet contains age-specific activities for students in the middle elementary grades. Some of the same activities in this program are in the K–2 program. However, in addition, sports and organized activities that are appropriate for the grade level have been added. The cognitive activities are more sophisticated and include reading books or stories, making lists, or writing about physical activity.

Slam Jammers—The "It's Your Move" Program for Grades 5–6: The Slam Jammers booklet contains age-specific activities for intermediate grade students. Many more independent activities and sports activities are included. The cognitive activities are more complex and involve report writing and data collection activities.

Students who complete 20 of the "It's Your Move" activities will add their names to the class poster of those completing the program. The goal is to have students encouraging each other to do lifestyle activities. Some suggestions for making the "It's Your Move" program successful in your school follow:

◆ **School program leader**—The program is most likely to be successful if one person in the school takes responsibility for the program. This person would contact The Prudential FITNESSGRAM or AAHPERD (see address and phone number in chapter 7) to obtain the program materials. This person would then have a meeting of teachers to explain program implementation. **The key is to communicate that the teachers will not have a lot of extra work if the program is implemented.** The teachers' responsibility is to distribute the booklets, briefly explain the program, and collect the booklets when completed. The students record their own names on the class chart provided. Incentives are available for school leaders.

◆ **Class discussion**—Class discussions of the various "It's Your Move" activities can be motivational. It is especially important to encourage out-of-school participation.

◆ **Parental involvement**—For the program to be successful, parental (or other adult) participation is essential. Presenting the "It's Your Move" program at a PTA/PTO or special physical fitness program will help participation. Direct contact with the parent almost always prompts greater participation.

◆ **Other suggestions**—Many of the ideas presented on the following pages for the Get Fit recognition program will be useful.

Get Fit:
A Program to Recognize Regular Physical Activity

The Get Fit recognition is given to any student who completes a 6-week exercise program. VA 2.7 describes the Get Fit exercises, and VA 2.8 gives the rules for earning recognition and includes a log for keeping track of progress. Some suggestions for implementing Get Fit follow:

◆ Copy VA 2.7 and VA 2.8 and give a copy to each student to take home.
◆ Demonstrate the Get Fit warm-up, workout, and cool-down exercises in one or two class periods.
◆ Explain the rules.
◆ Encourage students to take the program sheet home and put it on the refrigerator to make it easy to keep track of progress.
◆ Encourage students to try to get parents and other family members to exercise with them occasionally.
◆ Give weekly feedback in the form of stars or stickers to young students (ages 5–7). Ask students at the end of each week if they have done their exercises. If they have, give them a star or sticker to put in the margin by the week.

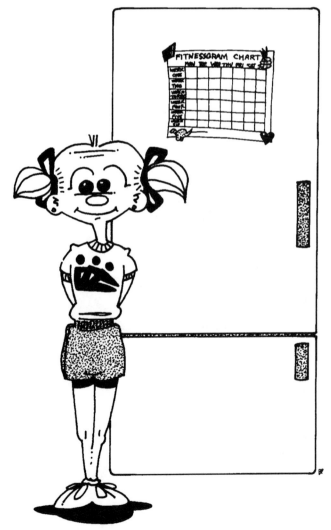

◆ Do the exercises in school periodically to reinforce them.
◆ Present the student with a Get Fit or a local fitness certificate when the signed completed log is returned. Sample certificates are available in The Prudential FITNESSGRAM *Test Administration Manual,* and one that can be reproduced is included as VA 5.5.
◆ Recognition can be done in class, at a Family Fitness Night, or at a recognition assembly.
◆ Post the names of those earning recognition on a bulletin board in the classroom or gymnasium.
◆ Encourage students to earn recognition more than once. When students do the program over and over again, they are learning and practicing the exercise behavior that leads to fitness improvement.
◆ Have students do the Get Fit program to prepare them to take The Prudential FITNESSGRAM test. Six weeks is required to

qualify for the Get Fit recognition. However, as few as 2 or 4 weeks will be of some benefit in preparing students to take the test.

Fit for Life:
A Program to Recognize Regular Physical Activity

This program is presented in VA 5.6. It can be copied, distributed, and taped to the refrigerator at home to encourage participation. It is excellent to use with older students. It gives them a chance to select their own activities and gives credit for participation in school and community sports programs. Students earn points from the point chart (shown in VA 5.6) over an 8-week period. Like Get Fit, it rewards regular participation and is possible to achieve by anyone who gives effort. Those who do the program will not only qualify for recognition but will also see improvements in fitness. Consider the same suggestions for this program as for the Get Fit program.

I'm Fit:
A Program to Recognize Physical Fitness Performance

Unlike the Get Fit and Fit for Life programs, I'm Fit recognizes students for the level of fitness attainment as well as their exercise behaviors. A student has to reach the Healthy Fitness Zone on at least four of the five tests to receive recognition. Because exercise behavior is critical to maintaining fitness, the student must also have earned "It's Your Move", Get Fit, or Fit for Life recognition or provide evidence of regular physical activity involvement (neighborhood, community, or school program).

The Prudential FITNESSGRAM Honor Recognition:
A Special Recognition Program

This program allows you to give any of The Prudential FITNESSGRAM recognitions to students who meet conditions of a contract arranged between you and the student. The recognition is excellent for special students, including those with special abilities or limiting disabilities. As the teacher, you may elect to recognize the participants with any of the recognition items (emblems, pins, painter's caps, or pencils) or with the special honor certificate. The recognition is designed to meet special needs. VA 5.7 is a sample contract that you can write with the student. Simply type or print the student's name and the conditions of the contract in the space provided (for example, take The Prudential FITNESSGRAM test two times, take home The Prudential FITNESSGRAM, and do "It's Your Move"). Have the student sign and date the contract, and you do the same. In some cases it may be necessary to consult with other teachers and parents in preparing the contract.

Local Fitness Recognition: A Special Recognition Program

This recognition is for those schools electing not to participate in the regular recognition programs of The Prudential FITNESSGRAM. You can set your own eligibility criteria and use the certificate provided (VA 5.5).

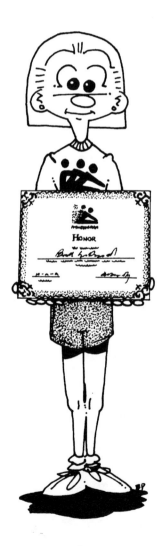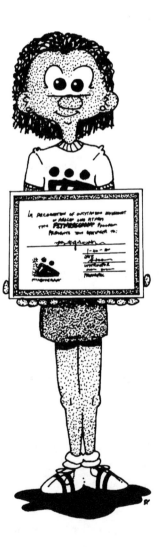

General Suggestions for Using the Recognition Program

Year-Long Exercise

Most fitness experts agree that regular exercise behavior is the key to building fitness and establishing lifetime exercise habits. The lack of fitness commonly attributed to American children is said to result from lack of activity outside the school. Physical education by itself cannot provide children with enough time to develop their physical fitness adequately. For this reason, a combination of fitness programs and recognition that encourages regular activity throughout the year is important. To start the year, the "It's Your Move" program should be encouraged. It is excellent for preparing for the fitness testing and provides 6 weeks of regular exercise. After completing the "It's Your Move" program, students may complete the Fit for Life or Get Fit programs. Students can be encouraged to repeat any of these more than once. Since the Fit for Life program includes many different activities, students can be encouraged to do different activities for points the second or third time the recognition is earned. Doing all of these programs would provide year-long activity.

Recognition for Year-Long Exercise

The Prudential FITNESSGRAM Honor Recognition could be designated for those who earn the "It's Your Move", Get Fit, and Fit for Life recognition at least once each. These requirements would assure many weeks of exercise during the school year.

School Charts

A school chart with a list of names of those who have earned recognition could be posted in the gym or school hallway. A special chart is included as part of the "It's Your Move" program.

Repeat Testing

Though "official" testing may be done only in the fall and spring, other testing can be done throughout the school year. It is not necessary that all tests be given at the same time. Also it is important that students begin to learn to test themselves. People will need to self-test when they are out of school if lifetime fitness is the goal.

Periodically, students can take each test in class. After an introduction is given, students can test themselves or work with a partner to obtain test results. Results can be recorded on a self-test reporting card (VA 3.1). The results can then be transferred to the Exercise and Fitness Log (VA 5.8a and b). In this way, students can keep track of fitness progress.

Recordkeeping

VA 5.8a and 5.8b can be used to keep year-long records. It allows students to keep track of exercise behavior and fitness changes. A record chart provides students with success feedback and can motivate continued participation. You may want to recognize fitness improvements that are accompanied by regular exercise participation. Results obtained from self-testing (see above) can be recorded with regular fall and spring testing on the recordkeeping chart. Some suggestions for using VA 5.8a and 5.8b, the Exercise and Fitness Log, are listed below.

◆ **Reproduce on card stock**—This will make the log more durable. Copy 5.8a on the front and 5.8b on the back of the same sheet.

◆ **Distribute to students**—Have them record their names and the school year. This should be done after the first testing of the year with The Prudential FITNESSGRAM . Record test results and the date of the tests on the card. Also have students fill in the fitness profile by copying the information from their Prudential FITNESSGRAM report card before they take it home.

◆ **Collect cards and file them**—Students may ask to add information at any time.

The Prudential FITNESSGRAM honor recognition would be an excellent reward for students who have kept records and show regular exercise as evidenced by completion of several programs and who have shown improvement on fitness as a result.

◆ **If a student earns recognition, he or she will write in the date and put an X over the box of the recognition earned**—The X should go over the #1 box for the first recognition. Boxes are provided for repeat recognition. If you have stickers, you may have younger students use these rather than X's.

◆ **If a student takes a test or all tests again, the results should be recorded again with the date.** The bar for each test should be filled in. The mark should be longer than the previous test if the score improved.

Fitness Clubs

Organization of a Fitness Club to do group activities before school, at lunch, at recess, or after school can be effective. Students can perform the Get Fit exercises and earn recognition together. The Fitness Club also provides an opportunity for students to find partners with whom they might earn Fit for Life recognition. Students can encourage each other to attend.

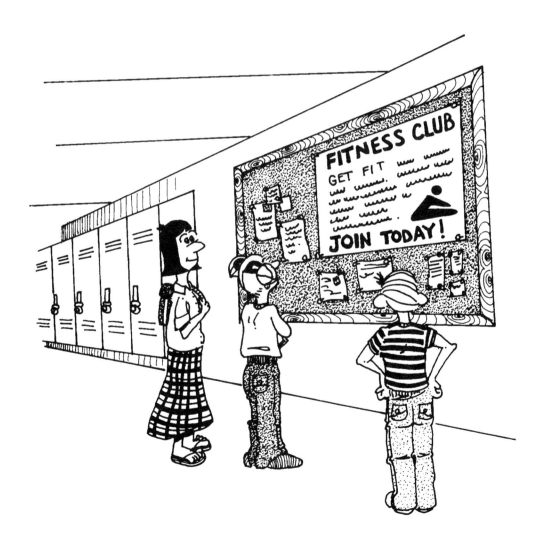

Family Fitness Nights

Family Fitness Nights are described in chapter 6. Recognition programs can be explained at a Family Fitness Night to urge parents to help students in earning fitness recognition.

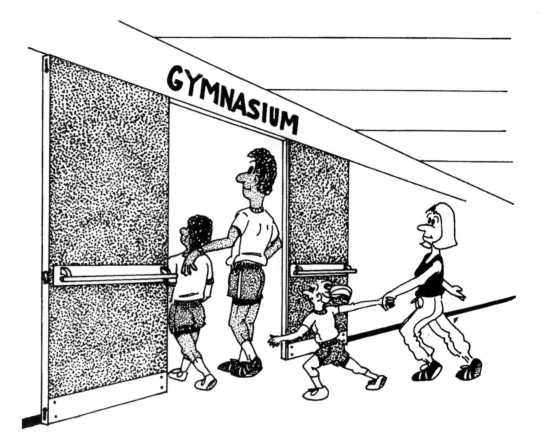

Funding the Recognition Program

The primary purpose of a recognition program should be to provide motivation to all students. Criteria for The Prudential FITNESSGRAM recognition have been established so that they are based on behavior and obtainable by most students. Therefore, you may find that more of your students will be eligible for recognition than in more traditional performance-based programs.

The items offered by The Prudential FITNESSGRAM have been selected to provide you a variety at prices sensitive to school budgets. If you find that your budget will not allow you to furnish items to the extent that you would like, you may wish to seek alternate sources of funding. Any of the following groups may be able to assist in providing recognition items for your students:

- PTA/PTO
- Community service clubs (Kiwanis, Rotary, Lions, etc.)
- Local businesses

Local businesses and service clubs are often quite interested in assisting with a school-related project, especially when it will impact students throughout the community. When approaching other organizations, be certain to explain the following concepts of The Prudential FITNESSGRAM:

- Health-related approach
- Comparison of students to standards rather than to each other
- Emphasis on development of exercise behavior rather than performance
- High probability for motivating all students with reasonable standards and goals.

Participation Incentives

A variety of items may be purchased for use in a motivation and recognition program using the form at the back of the book (see also chapter 7). In addition to these items, a blackline master of a certificate is provided (see VA 5.5) for teachers to make their own.

—6—
Family Fitness Activities

Testing students using The Prudential FITNESSGRAM is just the beginning of a total program to improve their fitness levels. Much more important than the results of the test is the ability to change their lifestyles. The Prudential FITNESSGRAM test is the first necessary step toward improved fitness. However, effective changes demand a total commitment from the family unit.

Most students are not in a position to control their diet or activity levels while at home. Parents may see homework, piano lessons, and cleaning the bedroom as important tasks but seldom take an active role in encouraging regular daily activity for their students. In most cases, if parents are unfit, their children will be unfit as well.

Many parents do not understand the physical capacities of their children. They are unaware of the level of physical work or activity that a student can reasonably be expected to accomplish. Parents generally do not perceive their children to be unfit. Adults usually regard children as healthy if they are not sick or complaining about their health. Unfortunately, a large number of our students are unfit and overweight. A Family Fitness Night can be a valuable technique for educating students and parents toward a better understanding of the need for regular activity by everyone.

Preparing for a Family Fitness Night

Adequate preparation is essential to ensure the success of an event such as a Family Fitness Night. The following steps are suggested in preparing for the event.

Medical Clearance

It should be made clear to parents that no one should participate in an activity that might aggravate a medical problem. An easy way to assess the activity readiness of parents is to administer the Par Q (VA 6.1). Make copies of the Par Q and distribute them to parents prior to the activity session. This will allow parents to assess whether they should actively participate in the evening's activities.

The activities enjoyed by the group should be noncompetitive and self-directed so that participants will not want to compete with others. Too often, this sense of competitiveness results in students and parents overexerting, only to discover sore muscles and stiff joints the next day. This results in a negative feeling about exercise and may lead to early burnout. Fitness is a personal matter, and parents and students should learn this lesson early in the session.

Publicity

Publicize the program well in advance so that as many parents as possible can attend. Distribute a take-home letter (VA 6.2) to the students, and put up posters throughout the school. Write a short press release about the program (VA 6.3) for the local newspaper or television station. Remind students in class to bring their parents. The more interest your session generates, the greater will be the credibility of the presentation.

Duration of Program

Limit the length of time that parents are required to participate. Thirty minutes is plenty of time on a school night. Most parents become bored with a program if it lasts longer than this.

Teaching Aids

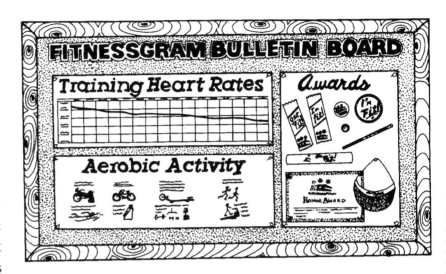

Take the opportunity to share various materials and information about your program at the Family Fitness Night. Dress up the gymnasium with attractive and informative bulletin boards. Training heart rates and aerobic activity are only two possible topics for bulletin boards. As part of the program, have students explain the information on the bulletin boards. Have a videotape machine playing which shows students in a typical physical education lesson. This is one of the few times that parents are a captive audience and can be educated about the worth of a physical education program.

Adopt a Program Format

It is desirable to develop a reputation for lively, fact-filled presentations. The following is suggested and may be modified as necessary.

◆ **Introduction and opener, 5 minutes**—This section should focus audience attention on the objectives of the evening's activities. It may be a handout which evaluates parents' activity attitudes and habits. It may be a brief discussion of reasons for performing different types of activities. It may be a discussion of the importance of fitness testing. In any case, the purpose is to prepare parents and students for the upcoming activity.

◆ **Warm-up activity, 5 minutes**—This section should involve participants in physical activity. The objective is to psychologically and physiologically prepare participants for activity. This activity might be some type of tag game, stretching activity, or personal challenge activity. It should be noncompetitive and focus on movement. It could include the warm-up activities in VA 2.17.

- ◆ **Fitness focus activity, 15 minutes**—This activity should be the fitness routine, self-testing program, or teaching presentation. This part of the program should be characterized by snappy, short, and concise segments of students in fitness activities. Parents come to view their own children and are admittedly bored when watching other children. A variety of activities utilizing children of all ages will result in a well-accepted program.
- ◆ **Cool-down, 5 minutes**—The cool-down activity should illustrate the need for gradually ending the workout to help the body return to normal. It should involve stretches and walking or slow jogging. Cooling down gradually can help prevent excessive muscle soreness. The cool-down can also be used as a quiet time to bring closure to the presentation.

Suggested Presentations

Presentation 1

Family Fitness Night

The Prudential FITNESSGRAM Self-Testing Program

- ◆ **Purpose**—This program will teach parents and students how to perform and interpret The Prudential FITNESSGRAM fitness test. Spinoffs from the program will be that parents can directly observe the fitness level of their children and leave with a better understanding of their personal fitness level. Since time will restrict this activity session, the one mile run/walk should be omitted from the testing. Parents may be encouraged to do the one-mile test at some other time. Set up a station near each corner of the gym and attach a copy of VAs 3.4–3.11 to each one. There should be four stations with enough equipment to test 6 to 8 participants simultaneously.

  It is recommended that The Prudential FITNESSGRAM promotional video be shown to provide parents with a general overview of The Prudential FITNESSGRAM program. Details on obtaining the video are provided in chapter 7.
- ◆ **Introduction and opener**—Hand out copies of VA 3.1 to facilitate recording the scores on the fitness test items: push-ups, curl-ups, back-saver sit-and-reach, and skinfold measurements. Briefly discuss that each station has a text explanation and the required equipment. See Figure 1 for information about setting up the four stations.
- ◆ **Warm-up**—Play Parent Group Tag for a warm-up. Every person must have at least one partner. A few sets of partners are designated as "it" and chase

Station 1: Curl-up Testing—
Tumbling mats, measuring strips
(see page 27), and a stop watch are
placed at this station.

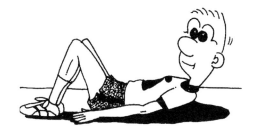

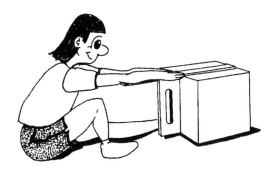

**Station 2: Back-Saver
Sit-and-Reach Testing—**
Sit-and-reach boxes are placed
at this station.

Station 3: Push-up Testing—
Stopwatches and mats are placed
at this station.

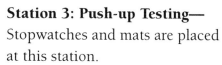

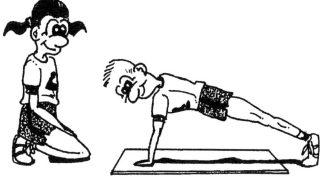

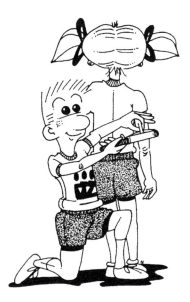

Station 4: Skinfold Measurements—
Calipers and boxes or a bench for foot
placement (for testing the calf skinfold)
are placed at this station.

Figure 1. Test item demonstration stations.

others. When those who are "it" tag another pair, that pair becomes "it," replacing the pair that tagged them. Adults must be paired with at least one partner who is a child. The size of the groups is not restricted. If any group releases their hand grip while being chased, they automatically become "it."

◆ **Fitness focus activity**—Divide parents and students into four equal size groups and move each group to a station. Parents and students test each other and record their scores on the scorecards (VA 3.1). A copy of VAs 2.5 and 2.6 can be given as a handout or used as posters placed at stations so parents and students can see what the minimum level of performance should be.

A variation of this activity is to set up a number of personal computers and use The Prudential FITNESSGRAM form to report test scores of the students. Parents can input the test scores of their children into the computer and receive a Prudential FITNESSGRAM report card to take home. Because The Prudential FITNESSGRAM software is designed for children, it is not possible to print a Prudential FITNESSGRAM for the parent.

◆ **Cool-down**—Spend the last few minutes of the session discussing the results of The Prudential FITNESSGRAM test. Concentrate on interpreting the results and explaining how to improve the fitness levels of all participants. A caution: try to avoid discussing personal problems or results. Concentrate on general statements and concerns. Personal matters should be discussed individually since they generally are not of interest to the rest of the group. A discussion of the various forms of recognition and how parents can help their children earn them could be included.

◆ **"It's Your Move" presentation**—If you plan to use "It's Your Move" with your students, a brief explanation and distribution of booklets directly to parents is a good idea. VA 5.1 to 5.4 could be used to help explain the program. This would be an excellent ending activity.

Presentation 2

School Fitness Night

◆ **Purpose**—The purpose of this presentation is to show parents the wide variety of fitness activities performed in the physical education program. Parents are invited to participate with their children and encouraged to use personal judgment in resting or refraining from activity when necessary.

◆ **Introduction and opener**—Distribute a handout which briefly describes the various fitness routines. Give the length of time the fitness activities are usually performed since only a short sample of each routine will be demonstrated. See chapter 4 for listings and descriptions of sample routines.

◆ **Warm-up**—All parents who want to participate are invited on the floor. Play an active game which involves all students in activity. See the section on Fitness Games (chapter 4, pp. xx–xx) for suggestions. Tag games are particularly effective since students (and parents, too) demonstrate a great deal of enthusiasm and excitement when playing. Play two or three games and move to the next section.

◆ **Fitness focus activity**—Have students demonstrate a wide variety of fitness activities. The purpose of the demonstration should be to show that the fitness routines exercise all body parts rather than to provide a strenuous workout session for the demonstration group. Each routine should be about 2 minutes in length, which will allow time for 7 to 8 routines. A great deal can be added to the presentation by having an announcer discuss how the routines are organized and why they were selected.

◆ **Cool-down**—Give parents and students 5 minutes to walk and ask questions about activities which have been performed. At various intervals, stop the group and lead them through stretches.

◆ **"It's Your Move"**—If you plan to use "It's Your Move" with your students, a brief explanation and distribution of booklets directly to parents is a good idea. VAs 5.1 to 5.4 could be used to help explain the program. This would be an excellent ending activity.

♦ **Questions and answers**—Complete the evening by answering questions. Caution must be used to assure that parents do not ask questions that are personal in nature, such as about their own children. Questions should be focused on topics such as importance of fitness, techniques, and duration and intensity of activity.

Presentation 3

Family Play-Together Night

♦ **Purpose**—The focus of this presentation is to show parents how they can become involved in fitness development activities with their children.

♦ **Opener**—Use VA 6.4 to check the family's attitude toward activity, nutrition, and wellness. Discuss the importance of understanding the need for fitness and having a positive familial attitude at home. Parents and students are involved in the activity.

♦ **Warm-up**—Rope-jumping activities are excellent since some type of rope is usually readily available. Begin the warm-up with a few easy stretches using a folded jump rope to stimulate the stretches. For example: Hold the folded jump rope overhead and twist the body at the hips back and forth. Hold the rope and touch the toes. Sit with the legs extended and put the folded rope near or past the feet. Continue the warm-up by jumping the rope to music. Encourage students and parents to demonstrate different ways of jumping the rope.

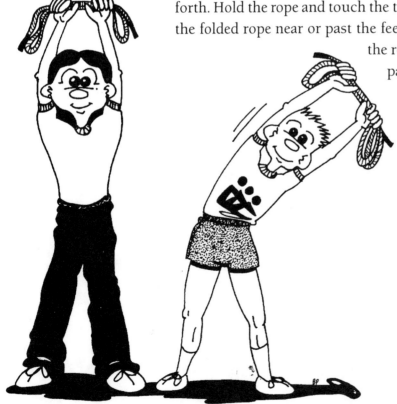

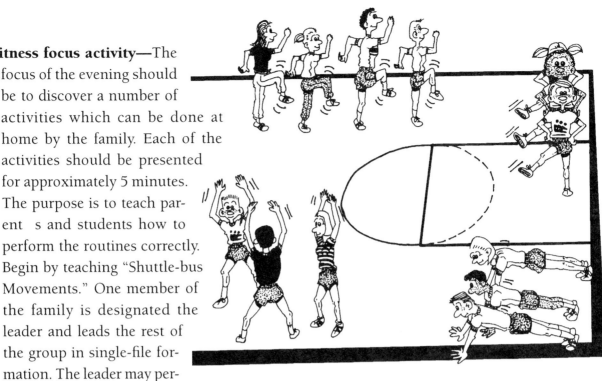

◆ **Fitness focus activity**—The focus of the evening should be to discover a number of activities which can be done at home by the family. Each of the activities should be presented for approximately 5 minutes. The purpose is to teach parent s and students how to perform the routines correctly. Begin by teaching "Shuttle-bus Movements." One member of the family is designated the leader and leads the rest of the group in single-file formation. The leader may perform any type of activity desired as long as he or she continues to move. On signal or at specified intervals, the leader moves to the end of the line and the next person leads the group activity. Any leader may stop and lead the group in a stretching or strength activity; however, only one of these activities should be performed consecutively.

The next activity is "Continuity Activities," which involves alternating rope jumping with exercises. Using an audiotape which has repeated intervals of 30 seconds of music followed by 30–45 seconds of silence is an excellent technique. When the music is playing, parents and students jump rope; when silence occurs, exercises are performed. Use a set of exercises which places demands on all parts of the body. VA 6.5 shows all the exercises in chapter 4 grouped according to the area of the body developed. Explain that parents should select at least two exercises from each group. In addition, consecutive exercises should not exercise the same body parts.

The next routine to be presented is "Aerobic Activity and Partner Resistance Exercises." Again, if desired, an audiotape with intervals of 30–45 seconds of music will signal the aerobic activity. When the silence interval (1–1.5 minutes) occurs, partner resistance exercises are performed. See chapter 4 for a description of aerobic activity and partner resistance exercises. The partner resistance exercises are a particularly good choice because they require a partner and encourage the parent and child to work together on fitness-oriented activities. Hand out VA 6.6, which shows how to perform aerobic activities and partner resistance exercises.

◆ **Cool-down**—"Follow the Leader Stretch and Move" is performed to allow parents and students to discuss activities. Discuss the basic purposes of a cooling-down period (helps the body return to normal after a workout and provides the opportunity to stretch muscles and develop flexibility).

Note: Announce that any person who feels he or she should not participate in specific activities should feel free to sit down during these activities.

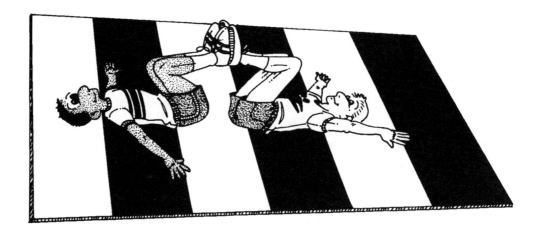

—7—

Resource Materials

Good information on health, fitness, and nutrition is available from many different sources.

The American Alliance for Health, Physical Education, Recreation and Dance and The Cooper Institute for Aerobics Research:
A Partnership to Promote Health-Related Fitness
In 1994, the American Alliance for Health, Physical Education, Recreation and Dance (AAHPERD) and the Cooper Institute for Aerobics Research (CIAR) established a partnership in support of health-related youth fitness. Under this agreement, both organizations will endorse, adopt, and promote AAHPERD's Physical Best educational materials and CIAR's The Prudential FITNESSGRAM testing program.

The American Alliance for Health, Physical Education, Recreation and Dance (AAHPERD), with over 29,000 members, is the leading professional association for health and physical educators. AAHPERD comprises six associations. It arranges hundreds of conferences, conventions, seminars, workshops, demonstrations, and symposia each year. In addition, AAHPERD publishes four periodicals and over 300 book titles on health, physical education, leisure, and dance. To find out more about AAHPERD publications, order a complementary copy of the AAHPERD catalog by calling 1-800-321-0789. For information on other AAHPERD programs, write or call AAHPERD, 1900 Association Drive, Reston, VA 22091. Phone: (703) 476-3400.

The Cooper Institute for Aerobics Research (CIAR) is an independent nonprofit organization active in research, public policy, and education relating to cardiovascular fitness and physical activity. Among CIAR's eight divisions, the Division of Childhood and Adolescent Health operates and delivers The Prudential FITNESSGRAM program. It provides products and technical assistance to the approximately 3,000 schools and agencies that use The Prudential FITNESSGRAM. The division also conducts research studies on issues relevant to the health of children and adolescents, including nutrition, injuries and violence, physical activity, and preventive cardiology. For more information, write or call: The Cooper Institute for Aerobics Research, 12330 Preston Road, Dallas, TX 74230, Phone (800) 635-7050.

Books

AAHPERD. 1987. *Basic Stuff Series.* AAHPERD Publications, P.O. Box 385, Oxon Hill, MD 20750-0385, FAX 301-567-9553.
   —*An excellent series for teaching concepts related to fitness.*

AAHPERD. 1989. *The Physical Best Educational Kit.* AAHPERD Publications, P.O. Box 385, Oxon Hill, MD 20750-0385, FAX 301-567-9553.
   —*A teaching kit that includes instructor's guide, teaching ideas cards, methods of integrating a recognition system, and reproducible samples of key elements of the Physical Best program.*

Althaus, R. A., Thompson, M., Walker, N., and Zuti, W. B. 1987. *Health.* Scott, Foresman and Co., 1900 E. Lake Blvd., Glenview, IL 60625.
   —*A health textbook for junior and senior high school students.*

Arnheim, D. D., and Sinclair, W. A. 1985. *Physical Education for Special Populations: A Developmental, Adapted, and Remedial Approach.* Englewood Cliffs, NJ: Prentice-Hall.
   —*A textbook with general information regarding adapting physical activities for students with disabilities.*

Bar-Or, O. 1983. *Pediatric Sports Medicine for the Practitioner.* New York: Springer-Verlag.
   —*A reference book containing information about children and exercise.*

Bennett, J., and Kamiya, A. 1987. *Fitness and Fun for Everyone.* Great Activities Publishing Company, P.O. Box 51158, Durham, NC 27717-1158, Phone: (919) 489-5990.
   —*Activities reference book containing many creative, motivating fitness activities.*

Cooper, K. H. 1982. *The Aerobics Program for Total Well-Being.* New York: Bantam Books.
   —*A general exercise and fitness reference book.*

Corbin, C. B. 1974. *Concepts of Fitness and Wellness,* 1st ed. Dubuque, IA: Brown/Benchmark, 2460 Kerper Blvd., Dubuque, IA 52001.
   —*A good resource book for teachers.*

Corbin, C. B., and Corbin, D. E. 1991. *Homemade Play Equipment,* 2nd ed. American Press, 520 Commonwealth Avenue, Boston, MA 02215.
   —*A reference book describing numerous pieces of equipment that can be constructed from readily available materials.*

Corbin, C. B., and Lindsey, R. 1993. *Fitness for Life,* 3rd ed. Scott, Foresman and Co., 1900 E. Lake Blvd., Glenview, IL 60625.
   —*A general fitness and exercise book.*

Corbin, C. B., and Lindsey, R. 1994. *Concepts of Physical Fitness,* 8th ed. Dubuque, IA; Brown/Benchmark, 2460 Kerper Blvd., Dubuque, IA 52001.
   —*Textbook for junior and senior high schools.*

Cratty, B. J. 1980. *Adapted Physical Education for Handicapped Children and Youth.* Denver, CO: Love Publishing Company.
   —*A textbook with general information regarding adapting physical activities for students with disabilities.*

Fait, H. F., and Dunn, J. M. 1982. *Special Physical Education: Adapted, Corrective, Developmental,* 5th ed. Philadelphia: W. B. Saunders Publishing.
   —*A textbook with general information regarding adapting physical activities for students with disabilities.*

Falls, H., Boyler, A., and Dishman, R. 1980. *Essentials of Fitness.* Philadelphia: W. B. Saunders Publishing.
   —*A general fitness and exercise reference book.*

Gym Dandies Quarterly. 1988–89. Great Activities Publishing Company, P.O. Box 51158, Durham, NC 27717-1158, Phone: (919) 489-5990.
   —*An activities reference manual published quarterly. Each publication emphasizes activities related to a specific area of the physical education curriculum.*

Gym Dandies, Volumes I and II. 1986–87; 1987–88. Great Activities Publishing Company, P.O. Box 51158, Durham, NC 27717-1158, Phone: (919) 489-5990.
   —*Bound reprints of the Gym Dandies Quarterly in two volumes (vol. 1, 1986–87; vol. 2, 1987–88). Each volume includes one section devoted to fitness activities.*

Hirst, C. C., and Michaelis, E. 1983. *Retarded Kids Need to Play.* Leisure Press, 597 Fifth Ave., New York, NY 10017.

Kamiya, A. 1985. *Elementary Teacher's Handbook of Indoor and Outdoor Games.* Parker Publishing, available through Great Activities Publishing Company, P.O. Box 51158, Durham, NC 27717-1158, Phone (919) 489-5990.
   —*A reference manual containing hundreds of games and activities, many of which can be used very effectively as fitness activities.*

Kravitz, Len. 1986. *Anybody's Guide to Total Fitness.* Dubuque, IA: Kendall/Hunt Publishing.
   —*General information and specific movement suggestions for aerobic dance activities.*

Kuntzleman, C. T. 1982. *Aerobics with Fun.* Fitness Finders, P.O. Box 160, Spring Arbor MI 49283-0160, Phone: (517) 750-1500.
   —*A reference book with over 1,100 activities for developing fitness in children.*

Kuntzleman, C. T. 1982. *Fitness for Junior High Students.* Fitness Finders, P.O. Box 160, Spring Arbor, MI 49283-0160, Phone: (517) 750-1500.
   —*A reference book with numerous routines for developing cardiovascular fitness (for use in conjunction with* Aerobics with Fun*).*

Pangrazi, R. P., and Hastad, D. N. 1989. *Physical Fitness in the Elementary Schools,* 2nd ed. AAHPERD Publications, P.O. Box 385, Oxon Hill, MD 20750-0385, FAX: (301) 567-9553.
   —*A reference book containing activities and ideas for stimulating fitness in K–6 grade children.*

Pangrazi, R. P., and Darst, P. W. 1991. *Dynamic Physical Education for Secondary School Students,* 2nd ed. Macmillan Distributing Center, Attn: Order Department, 100 Front Street, Riverside NJ 08075, Phone: (800) 323-7445.
  —*A textbook containing many fitness routines and wellness activities for junior and senior high school students.*

Pangrazi, R. P., and Dauer, V. P. 1995. *Dynamic Physical Education for Elementary School Children,* 11th ed. Boston: Allyn and Bacon. To order: The Education Company, 2949 Linus Way, Carmichael, CA 95608, Phone: (916) 483-8846.
  —*A textbook with fitness activities and active games for elementary school children.*

Pangrazi, R. P., and Dauer, V. P. 1995. *Lesson Plans for Dynamic Physical Education for Elementary School Children,* 11th ed. Boston: Allyn and Bacon. To order: The Education Company, 2949 Linus Way, Carmichael, CA 95608, Phone: (916) 483-8846.
  —*A year-long set of weekly lesson plans for teaching a comprehensive physical education program.*

Pollock, M. L., Wilmore, J. K., and Fox, S. M. 1984. *Exercise in Health and Disease.* Philadelphia: W. B. Saunders Publishing.
  —*A general fitness and exercise reference book.*

Richmond, J. B., Pounds, E. T., and Corbin, C. B. 1990. *Health for Life.* Scott, Foresman, and Co., 1900 E. Lake Blvd., Glenview, IL 60625.
  —*A series of textbooks, one for each grade level K–8. Each contains chapters on exercise, fitness, and nutrition.*

Sherrill, C. 1986. *Adapted Physical Education and Recreation: A Multi-disciplinary Approach,* 3rd ed. Dubuque, IA: Wm. C. Brown Co.
  —*Basic information regarding many disabilities that provides suggestions for adapting activities.*

Stillwell, J., and Stockard, J. 1988. *More Fitness Exercises for Children.* Great Activities Publishing Company, P.O. Box 51185, Durham, NC 27717-1158, Phone: (919) 489-5990.

Van Gelder, N., and Marks, S. (Eds.). 1987. *Aerobic Dance Exercise Instructor Manual.* International Dance Exercise Association Foundation, 2431 Morena Blvd., Suite 2D, San Diego, CA 92110, Phone: (619) 275-1881.
—*General information and specific movement suggestions for aerobic dance activities.*

Winnick, J. P., and Short, F. X. 1985. *Physical Fitness Testing of the Disabled: Project UNIQUE.* Human Kinetics Publishers, P.O. Box 5076, Champaign, IL 61825-5076, Phone: (800) DIAL-HKP.
—*Presents information on levels of performance on fitness measures for individuals with disabilities.*

Articles

AAHPERD. 1991. Physical education and the public health: *RQES* Forum. *Research Quarterly for Exercise and Sport, 63,* 295–333.
—*Seven articles by leading experts in the field of youth fitness.*

AAHPERD. 1992. Are children and youth fitness? *RQES* Forum. *Research Quarterly for Exercise and Sport, 62,* 123–151.
—*Five articles on the role of physical education in the public health.*

AAHPERD. National children and youth fitness study results. 1. Results for young children. *JOPERD,* December, 1987, 50–102. 2. Results for older youth. *JOPERD,* January, 1985 (special insert), 1–48.
—*The results of the fitness study appear in two issues of* JOPERD. *Each issue contains several articles.*

Baranowski, T., et al. 1992. Assessment, prevalence, and cardiovascular benefits of physical activity and fitness in youth, *Medicine and Science in Sports and Exercise, 24*(6S), S237–247.

Blair, S. N. 1993. 1993 C. H. McCloy Research Lecture: Physical activity, physical fitness, and health. *Research Quarterly for Exercise and Sport, 64,* 365–376.

Blair, S. N., et al. 1989. Physical fitness and all-cause mortality: A prospective study of healthy men and women. *Journal of the American Medical Association, 262*(17), 2395–2401.

Blair, S. N., Kohl, H. W., and Gordon, N. F. 1992. Physical activity and
health: A lifestyle approach. *Medicine, Exercise, Nutrition, and Health, 1*,
54–57.

Bouchard, C. 1993. Heredity and health-related fitness. *Physical Activity and
Fitness Research Digest, 1*(4), 1–8.

Bunk, C. 1980. Muscle of the week. *JOHPER, 51*(7), 79.
—*Elementary program idea for teaching about muscles.*

Corbin, C. B. 1978. Changing consumers means new concepts. *JOPERD,
49*(1), 43.
—*How to teach concepts in secondary schools.*

Corbin, C. B. 1986. Fitness is for children: Developing lifetime fitness.
JOPERD, 57, 82–84.

Corbin, C. B. 1987. Physical fitness in the K–12 curriculum: Some defensible
solutions to perennial problems. *JOPERD, 58*, 49–54.

Corbin, C. B., and Laurie, D. R. 1978. Exercise for a lifetime: An educational
effort. *The Physician and Sportsmedicine, 6*, 51–55.
—*Teaching students to make meaningful decisions about exercise and
fitness for a lifetime.*

Corbin, C. B., and Pangrazi, R. P. 1992. Are American children and youth fit?
Research Quarterly for Exercise and Sport, 63, 96–106.

Corbin, C. B., and Pangrazi, R. P. 1993. The health benefits of physical
activity. *Physical Activity and Fitness Research Digest, 1*(1), 1–8.

Corbin, C. B., Whitehead, J. R., and Lovejoy, P. Y. 1988: Youth physical
fitness awards. *Quest, 40*(3), 302–218.

Cureton, K. J., and Warren, G. L. 1990. Criterion-referenced standards for
youth health-related fitness tests: A tutorial. *Research Quarterly for
Exercise and Sport, 61*, 7–19.

Edington, D. W., and Cunningham, L. 1973. Applied physiology of exercise:
A biological awareness concept. *JOHPER, 44*(8), 30–31.
—*Suggestions for teaching basic exercise physiology in elementary school
physical education.*

Gilliam, T. B., et al. 1982. Exercise programs for children: A way to prevent heart disease. *The Physician and Sportsmedicine, 10*, 98–100.

Johnston, J. G. 1980. Fun in fitness at the elementary school level. *Canadian Association for Health, Physical Education and Recreation Journal, 46*(2), 28–37.
—*Ideas to stimulate fitness in elementary school children.*

Lawson, H. A., and Lawson, B. 1977. An alternative program model for secondary school physical education. *JOHPER, 48*(7), 38–39.
—*Physical education programming that emphasizes conceptual learning.*

Levitt, S. L. 1980. Fitness on your own time. *JOHPER, 51*(9), 79–80.
—*Ideas for after-school fitness assignments.*

Meredith, M. D. 1988. Activity or fitness: Is the process or the product more important to public health? *Quest, 40*(3), 180–186.

Pangrazi, R. P., and Corbin, C. B. 1993. Physical fitness: Questions teachers ask. *JOPERD, 64*(7), 14–19.

Park, R. J. (no date). Measurement of physical fitness: A historical perspective, *ODPHP Monograph Series*, 1–37.

Pate, R. R. 1983. A new definition of fitness. *The Physician and Sportsmedicine, 11*, 77–80.

Pate, R. R. 1988. The evolving definition of fitness. *Quest, 40*(3), 174–179.

Placek, J. H. 1983. A conceptually-based physical education program. *JOPERD, 54*(7), 27–28.
—*High school program that teaches concepts during 9th grade and provides electives during 10th and 11th grades.*

Sallis, J. F., and McKenzie, T. L. 1991. Physical education's role in public health. *Research Quarterly for Exercise and Sport, 62*, 124–137.

Sallis, J. F., et al. 1992. Determinants of physical activity and interventions in youth. *Medicine and Science in Sports and Exercise, 24*(6S), S248–257.

Simons-Morton, B. G., Parcel, G. S., O'Hara, N. M., Blair, S. N., and Pate, R. R. 1988. Health-related physical fitness in childhood: Status and recommendations. *Annual Review of Public Health, 9,* 403–425.

Spindt, G. 1985. Fitness is basic. *JOPERD, 56*(7), 68–69.
   —*Description of a junior-high program that focuses on fitness improvement and conceptual understanding.*

Whitehead, J. R. 1993. Physical activity and intrinsic motivation, *Physical Activity and Fitness Research Digest, 1*(2), 1–8.

Audiovisual Materials

AAHPERD, 1900 Association Drive, Reston, VA 22091. Phone: (800) 476-2401.

Physical Best: Integrating Concepts with Activities (K–6 or 6–12) provides innovative ideas for enhancing fitness in a physical education program.

Skinfold Video teaches the techniques for measuring body fat using skinfolds.

American Heart Association, 7272 Greenville Ave., Dallas, TX 75231, Phone: (214) 373-6300, or contact the American Heart Association office listed in the white pages of the telephone book.

Lower Elementary Videotape (½ inch and ¾ inch) includes four films to use with the "Getting to Know Your Heart" package: *It's a Heart, Adventures of a Man in Search of a Heart, The Heart That Changed Color,* and *Dr. Truso's Jet Powered Pedaler.*

Upper Elementary Videotape (½ inch and ¾ inch) combines five films to use with the "Getting to Know Your Heart" package: *The Earthling Heart, Case of the Sudden Sickness, Heart Health for Fun, Who Killed Eldon Finney?* and *Who's in Charge?*

Health Education Videotape: Secondary (½ inch and ¾ inch) combines four films for adolescents: *Let's Talk About Smoking, Body Fuel, The Exercise Film,* and *What Goes Up.*

Circulation of the Blood, 16-mm film explains blood circulation through the body.

The Exercise Film, 16-mm film explains the benefits of and ways to build aerobic capacity.

Laurie, D., and Corbin, C. B. Teaching Lifetime Fitness. 1994. Available from Audio Visual Design, 2208 Fort Riley Blvd., Manhattan, KS 66502, Phone: (913) 539-1555.
—Ten video programs for teaching physical fitness concepts.
1. *Climbing the Fitness Stairway*
2. *Introduction to Physical Fitness*
3. *Preparing for Exercise*
4. *Fitness, Exercise and Good Health*
5. *How Much Is Enough?*
6. *Cardiovascular Fitness*
7. *Building Cardiovascular Fitness*
8. *Muscle Fitness*
9. *Flexibility*
10. *Body Fatness*

Lohman, T. *Measuring Body Fat Using Skinfolds.* 1988. Human Kinetics Videos, P.O. Box 5076, Champaign, IL 61820, Phone: (217) 351-5076.

Pangrazi, R. P., and Dauer, V. P. 1981. *Dynamic Physical Education for Elementary School Students.* New York: Macmillan Publishing Co.
—*Videotape demonstrating a comprehensive physical education program.*

Free and Inexpensive Materials

American Health Foundation, Know Your Body, 320 East 43rd Street, New York, NY 10017, Phone: (212) 953-1900.
—*A variety of fitness literature.*

American Heart Association, 7272 Greenville Ave., Dallas, TX 75231, Phone: (214) 373-6300, or contact the local American Heart Association office listed in the white pages of the telephone book.

Program Packages—instructional programs generally containing teacher's guide, posters, audiovisuals, and student resources.
- *Heart Treasure Chest (3–5 years)*
- *Getting to Know Your Heart (Lower and Upper)*
- *Heart Challenge (Junior and Senior High School)*

Activity Kits—fitness activity instructional units.
  - *Jump for the Heath of It, Basic Skills*
  - *Jump for the Health of It, Intermediate Single and Double Dutch Skills*
  - *The FITT Kit*
  - *Racing with the Wind*
  - *Heart Trivia Challenge, (Elementary and Secondary)*
  - *Heart Star*
  - *Active Pursuit, No Trivial Matter*
  - *Heart Trivia Challenge*
  - *Jump Rope for Heart*

Teacher Resources
  - *What Every Teacher Should Know by Heart*
  - *Putting Your Heart into the Curriculum, Junior (grades 7–9 and 10–12)*
  - *National Examination of Cardiovascular Knowledge*

Kellogg Company, Project Nutrition, P.O. Box 9113, St. Paul, MN 55191, Phone: (612) 474-1163.
  —*Offers a number of activities for teaching nutrition skills.*

Kellogg Company, Kellogg's Fitness Focus, P.O. Box 2599, One Kellogg Square, Battle Creek, MI 49016-3599, Phone: (616) 961-2000.
  —*Activities and teacher's guide for fitness instruction, grades 5–9.*

McDonald's Corporation, Consumer Affairs Department, McDonald's Plaza, Oakbrook, IL 60521, Phone (708) 575-3000.
  —*Action packets and films to aid nutrition and fitness instruction.*

National Dairy Council, 9360 Castlegate Drive, Indianapolis, IN 46256, Phone: (317) 842-3060.
  —*A wide variety of materials including posters and resource guides for teaching nutrition and fitness skills.*

President's Council on Physical Fitness and Sports, 701 Pennsylvania Avenue NW, Room 250, Washington, DC 20004, Phone: (202) 272-3421.
  —*A wide variety of informative materials dealing with various aspects of fitness.*

Shawnee Mission Public Schools, Sunflower Project. Mohawk Instructional Center, 6649 Lamar, Shawnee Mission, KS 66202.
  —*Educational materials dealing with cardiovascular health.*

Special Educators Press, P.O. Box 24240, Los Angeles, CA 90024.
   —*A wide variety of materials for teaching children with disabilities in various settings.*

U.S. Government Printing Office, Superintendent of Documents, P.O. Box 371954, Pittsburgh, PA 15250-7954. Phone (202) 783-3238.
   —*Write or call to receive a list of inexpensive publications dealing with health and physical fitness.*

Sources for Equipment

Cosom Equipment Corporation, P.O. Box 1426, Minneapolis, MN 55440
   —*Offers a wide variety of plastic and foam equipment.*

Fat Control, Inc., P.O. Box 10117, Towson, MD 21204, Phone: (301) 296-1993 (301) 830-2378
   —*Plastic adipometers for measuring skinfold.*

The Prudential FITNESSGRAM, Cooper Institute for Aerobics Research, 12330 Preston Rd., Dallas, TX 74230, Phone: (800) 635-7050
   —*Plastic adipometers for measuring skinfold.*

Flaghouse, 18 W. 18th Street, New York, NY 10011
   —*All types of equipment and supplies.*

J. E. Gregory, Inc., P.O. Box 3483, Spokane, WA 92220
   —*Wide variety of balls, beanbags, and jump ropes.*

GSC Athletic Equipment, 600 N. Pacific Avenue, San Pedro, CA 90733
   —*All types of equipment and supplies.*

NOVEL Products, Inc., P.O. Box 408, Rockton, IL 61072-0408
   —*Calipers, crunch-ster for testing curl-ups, and other fitness products.*

Ross Laboratories, Consumer Relations, Columbus, OH 43216, Phone: (614) 624-7677.
   —*Physical growth NCHS percentiles for boys and girls, ages 2–18 years*

Robert Widen Co., P.O. Box 2075, Prescott, AZ 86302
—*Wide variety of quality equipment, supplies, and apparatus. Equipment field-tested on regular basis.*

Shield Manufacturing, 425 Fillmore Avenue, Tonawanda, NY 14150
—*Plastic and foam fitness and sport equipment.*

Things from Bell, Inc., P.O. Box 706, Cortland, NY 13045
—*Variety of equipment and supplies.*

U.S. Games, 2116 Falling Leaf Circle, Brea, CA 92621, Phone: (714) 990-6075.
—*Physical education equipment that is developmentally appropriate for all ages.*

Wolverine Sports, Box 1941, Ann Arbor, MI 48106
—*Wide variety of equipment and supplies.*

— 8 —
Visual Aids and Handouts

In this chapter you will find 58 blackline copy masters, called Visual Aids (VA). These are referred to throughout the book. Each VA has a number so that it may be located easily in this chapter. Permission is granted to reproduce these masters for use in class. They can be used to make overhead transparencies or can be reproduced for handouts.

Overhead Transparencies

The blackline master can be reproduced on plastic using most modern copy machines. The plastic sheets (transparencies) made from the masters can be used as a visual aid with an overhead projector. If your school or organization does not have a machine for making plastic overhead transparencies, most copy centers now have machines for this purpose; for a few cents you can have an overhead transparency created. Some suggestions for reproduction and use are listed below.

You may want to use magic markers to color the transparency. Simply color the transparency in the desired areas using colored magic markers. You may have students make transparencies and color them as a part of a project. You can also encourage students to make presentations to the class using transparencies.

Some older copy machines will not make good transparencies directly from the masters in this book because they require a high carbon level in the master. If you have poor results, you can improve the quality of the transparency by first copying the master on a copying machine and then creating the transparency from the copy.

In elementary schools, the visual aids can be used in health or physical education class. Classroom and physical education teachers may want to work together for this instruction. If there is a school nurse, an ongoing nurse–teacher instructional effort is encouraged. In secondary schools, the visual aids may be used in regular physical education classes, in health or science classes, or in special Fitness for Life units.

The visual aids can also be used for special fitness programs for parents, to present fitness speeches to local groups, and to make presentations to school boards, scouting groups, and recreation–sports groups who are interested in fitness.

Handouts

Another way to use the blackline masters is to reproduce them as handouts. This can be done by copying them directly on a copying machine or by preparing copy masters for making multiple copies. If you are going to distribute large numbers, the copy master procedure is least expensive. As with transparencies, many modern machines will reproduce masters that can be used with ditto or mimeo machines. If you have a ditto or mimeo machine but no machine for creating a master, you can have masters made at most copy centers. Many suggestions for using handouts are discussed throughout this book; some of these uses are briefly reviewed here.

In-class work sheets—The handouts can be given to students to be used in class. They can be used as a basis for discussion. In some cases, they can be used as part of student projects.

Homework sheets—The handouts can be distributed with directions. The assignments can be done at home and returned.

Information to parents—The handouts can be sent home to parents for informational purposes. The Get Fit and Fit for Life program sheets not only provide information for parents but offer opportunities for parents to encourage regular activity among their children.

Personal information—Many of the sheets are merely to provide personal information to students to help them better understand fitness and exercise concepts and to motivate them to be active and fit.

Class projects—Handouts can be kept in a folder or envelope and submitted as part of a class project.

In VA 3.12, 6.2, and 6.3, spaces have been provided to allow the insertion of school name, teacher name, or date as appropriate to complete the information presented.

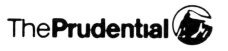 **The Prudential** **FITNESS**GRAM

COMMITTED TO HEALTH RELATED FITNESS
Developed by The Cooper Institute for Aerobics Research
Endorsed by The American Alliance for Health, Physical Education, Recreation and Dance

Jane Jogger
FITNESSGRAM Jr. High
FITNESSGRAM Test District

Instructor: Bridgman   Gregg
Grade: 04   **Period:** 09   **Age** 09

Test Date	Height	Weight
MO - YR	FT - IN	LBS
10.92	5.00	101
05.93	5.01	106

AEROBIC CAPACITY

HEALTHY FITNESS ZONE

One Mile Walk/Run

Needs Improvement	Good		Better
* * * * * * * * * * * * * *	* * * * * * *		
* * * * * * * * * * * * * * *	* * * * * * *		

10:00   07:30

Max VO$_2$ Indicates ability to use oxygen. Expressed as ml of oxygen per kg body weight per minute. Healthy Fitness Zone = 35+ for girls & 42+ for boys.

	Current	Past
	min:sec	
	9:01	9:12
	ml/kg	
	47	47

MUSCLE STRENGTH, ENDURANCE & FLEXIBILITY

HEALTHY FITNESS ZONE

Curl-up (Abdominal)

Needs Improvement	Good	Better
* * * * * * *		
* * * * * *		

21   40

# performed	
12	05

Push-up (Upper Body)

Needs Improvement	Good	Better

12   25

# performed	
27	20

Trunk Lift (Trunk Extension)

Needs Improvement	Good	Better

9   12

inches	
10	10

The test of flexibility is optional. If given, it is scored pass or fail and is performed on the right and left.

Test given: Back Saver Sit and Reach

Right	P
Left	P

BODY COMPOSITION

HEALTHY FITNESS ZONE

Percent Body Fat

Needs Improvement	Good	Better
* * * * * * * * * * *		
* * * * * * * * * *		

25.0   10.0

% fat	
27.0	31.1

You can improve your abdominal strength with curl-ups 2 to 4 times a week. Remember your knees are bent and no one holds your feet.

Your upper body strength was very good. Try to maintain your fitness by doing strengthening activities at least 2 03 3 times each week.

To improve your body composition, Joe, extend the length of vigorouse activity each day and follow a balanced nutritional program, eating more fruits and vegetables and fewer fats and sugars. Improving body composition may also help improve your other fitness scores.

Your aerobic capacity is in the Healthy Fitness Zone. Maintain your fitness by doing 20 - 30 minutes of vigorous activity at least 3 or 4 times each week.

To parent or guardian: The Prudential FITNESSGRAM is a valuable tool in assessing a young person's fitness level. The area of the bar highlighted in yellow indicates the "healthy fitness zone." All children should strive to maintain levels of fitness within the "healthy fitness zone" or above. By maintaining healthy fitness level for these areas of fitness your child may have a reduced risk for developing heart disease, obesity or low back pain. Some children may have personal interests that require higher levels of fitness (e.g. athletes).

Recommended activities for improving fitness are based on each individual's test performance. Ask your child to demonstrate each test item for you. Some teachers may stop the test when performance equals the upper limit of the "healthy fitness zone" rather than requiring a maximal effort.

Developing good exercise habits is important to maintaining lifelong health. You can help your son or daughter develop these habits by encouraging regular participation in physical activitiy.

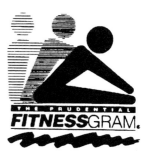

Sponsored by
The Prudential
Insurance Company
of America

VA 1.1

Total Fitness

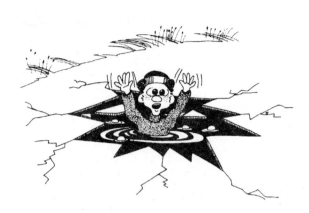

◆ *Meet Emergencies*

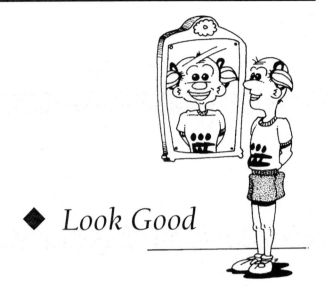

◆ *Look Good*

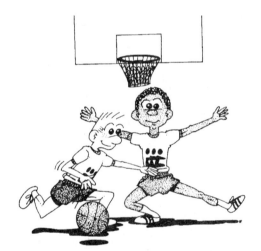

◆ *Enjoy Free Time*

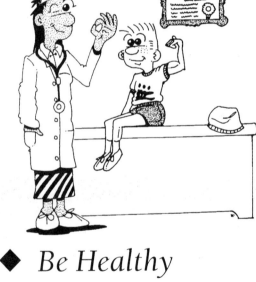

◆ *Be Healthy*

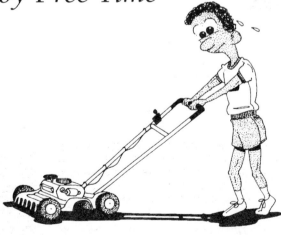

◆ *Work Efficiently*

VA 2.1

Fitness Areas

◆ *Aerobic Capacity*

◆ *Muscular Strength*

◆ *Muscular Endurance*

◆ *Body Composition*

◆ *Flexibility*

Why Do Fitness Tests?

- ◆ *Health Standards*

- ◆ *Fitness Needs*

- ◆ *Fitness Improvement*

- ◆ *Exercise Benefits*

Low Aerobic Capacity

Greater Risk of
—Heart Disease

Low Muscular Strength, Muscular Endurance, and Flexibility

Greater Risk of
—Back Pain
—Poor Posture
—Muscle Soreness
—Muscle Injury

Very Low Body Fat

Greater Risk of
—Eating Disorders
—Illness
—Slow Growth
of Vital Tissues
Such as Muscle
and Bone

Very High Body Fat

Greater Risk of
—Heart Disease
—Diabetes
—Hypertension
—Other Illnesses

Needs Improvement	*Healthy Fitness Zone*
Good	**Better**

VA 2.4

Table 2. The Prudential FITNESSGRAM
Standards for Healthy Fitness Zone*

BOYS

	One Mile (min:sec)		PACER (# laps)		V̇O₂max (ml/kg/min)		Percent Fat		Body Mass Index		Curl-up (# completed)	
5	*Completion of distance. Time standards not recommended.*		*Participate in run. Lap count standards not recommended.*				25	10	20	14.7	2	10
6							25	10	20	14.7	2	10
7							25	10	20	14.9	4	14
8							25	10	20	15.1	6	20
9							25	10	20	15.2	9	24
10	11:30	9:00	17	55	42	52	25	10	21	15.3	12	24
11	11:00	8:30	23	61	42	52	25	10	21	15.8	15	28
12	10:30	8:00	29	68	42	52	25	10	22	16.0	18	36
13	10:00	7:30	35	74	42	52	25	10	23	16.6	21	40
14	9:30	7:00	41	80	42	52	25	10	24.5	17.5	24	45
15	9:00	7:00	46	85	42	52	25	10	25	18.1	24	47
16	8:30	7:00	52	90	42	52	25	10	26.5	18.5	24	47
17	8:30	7:00	57	94	42	52	25	10	27	18.8	24	47
17+	8:30	7:00	57	94	42	52	25	10	27.8	19.0	24	47

	Trunk Lift (inches)		Push-up (# completed)		Modified Pull-up (# completed)		Pull-up (# completed)		Flexed Arm Hang (seconds)		Back Saver Sit & Reach** (inches)	Shoulder Stretch
5	6	12	3	8	2	7	1	2	2	8	8	Passing = Touching the fingertips together behind the back.
6	6	12	3	8	2	7	1	2	2	8	8	
7	6	12	4	10	3	9	1	2	3	8	8	
8	6	12	5	13	4	11	1	2	3	10	8	
9	6	12	6	15	5	11	1	2	4	10	8	
10	9	12	7	20	5	15	1	2	4	10	8	
11	9	12	8	20	6	17	1	3	6	13	8	
12	9	12	10	20	7	20	1	3	10	15	8	
13	9	12	12	25	8	22	1	4	12	17	8	
14	9	12	14	30	9	25	2	5	15	20	8	
15	9	12	16	35	10	27	3	7	15	20	8	
16	9	12	18	35	12	30	5	8	15	20	8	
17	9	12	18	35	14	30	5	8	15	20	8	
17+	9	12	18	35	14	30	5	8	15	20	8	

*Number on left is lower end of HFZ; number on right is upper end of HFZ
**Test scored Pass/Fail; must reach this distance to pass.

Table 3. The Prudential FITNESSGRAM
Standards for Healthy Fitness Zone*

GIRLS

	One Mile (min:sec)		PACER (# laps)		VO₂max (ml/kg/min)		Percent Fat		Body Mass Index		Curl-up (# completed)	
5	Completion of		Participate in				32	17	21	16.2	2	10
6	distance. Time		run. Lap count				32	17	21	16.2	2	10
7	standards not		standards not				32	17	22	16.2	4	14
8	recommended.		recommended.				32	17	22	16.2	6	20
9							32	17	23	16.2	9	22
10	12:30	9:30	7	35	39	47	32	17	23.5	16.6	12	26
11	12:00	9:00	9	37	38	46	32	17	24	16.9	15	29
12	12:00	9:00	13	40	37	45	32	17	24.5	16.9	18	32
13	11:30	9:00	15	42	36	44	32	17	24.5	17.5	18	32
14	11:00	8:30	18	44	35	43	32	17	25	17.5	18	32
15	10:30	8:00	23	50	35	43	32	17	25	17.5	18	35
16	10:00	8:00	28	56	35	43	32	17	25	17.5	18	35
17	10:00	8:00	34	61	35	43	32	17	26	17.5	18	35
17+	10:00	8:00	34	61	35	43	32	17	27.3	18.0	18	35

	Trunk Lift (inches)		Push-up (# completed)		Modified Pull-up (# completed)		Pull-up (# completed)		Flexed Arm Arm Hang (seconds)		Back Saver Sit & Reach** (inches)	Shoulder Stretch
5	6	12	3	8	2	7	1	2	2	8	9	
6	6	12	3	8	2	7	1	2	2	8	9	
7	6	12	4	10	3	9	1	2	3	8	9	
8	6	12	5	13	4	11	1	2	3	10	9	
9	6	12	6	15	4	11	1	2	4	10	9	Passing = Touching the fingertips together behind the back.
10	9	12	7	15	4	13	1	2	4	10	9	
11	9	12	7	15	4	13	1	2	6	12	10	
12	9	12	7	15	4	13	1	2	7	12	10	
13	9	12	7	15	4	13	1	2	8	12	10	
14	9	12	7	15	4	13	1	2	8	12	10	
15	9	12	7	15	4	13	1	2	8	12	12	
16	9	12	7	15	4	13	1	2	8	12	12	
17	9	12	7	15	4	13	1	2	8	12	12	
17+	9	12	7	15	4	13	1	2	8	12	12	

*Number on left is lower end of HFZ; number on right is upper end of HFZ
**Test scored Pass/Fail; must reach this distance to pass.

FITNESSGRAM
Get Fit Exercises

WARM-UP ACTIVITIES

Side Bend Trunk Twist Knee Lift Calf Stretch Arm Circles Jumping Jacks Brisk Walking Single Leg Lift Lunges Climbing Activities Arm/Side Stretch

STRENGTH DEVELOPMENT ACTIVITIES

Crunch Curl-ups Sit-ups Back Arch Wall Sit Push-ups Arm Curls Military Press (using canned food as weight) Modified Pull-ups Horizontal Ladder Activities

AEROBIC ACTIVITIES

Jogging Cycling Swimming Brisk Walking Rope Jumping Soccer Basketball

COOL-DOWN ACTIVITIES

Calf Stretch Thigh Stretch Sitting Toe Touch Knee Hug Arm/Shoulder Stretch

The Prudential FITNESSGRAM Get Fit Program

The Get Fit recognition can be earned by completing the recommended 6-week conditioning program. Each student should complete the exercise log below as evidence of participation in the activities and return the log to his or her teacher.

Get Fit rules are as follows:

1. Participation in the recommended Get Fit exercise program must be a minimum of 3 times each week for a 6-week period.
2. The participant should complete the exercise log and return it to his or her teacher. Teachers will verify participation and certify the student as eligible for the recognition.
3. In the event of illness or family emergency, the time period for earning the recognition may be extended according to the length of illness or emergency.
4. Exercise done as part of physical education or practice for participation on a sports team may substitute for one of the required three days.
5. In completing the exercise log, the student should indicate the dates for the week and place a check in the box for each day he or she completed a workout that included a warm-up, strength development activities, aerobic activities, and a cool-down.

Warm-up (WU)—At the beginning of a workout, perform three warm-up exercises from the suggested group or personal favorites. The activity should be at a slow, easy pace. Stretching exercises should be held for a count of 10. Do not bounce when stretching. Warm-up exercises should work the upper body and the legs.

Strength Development (SD)—Perform three strength development exercises each day from the suggested group or personal favorites. Perform the exercise as many times as you can up to 15.

Aerobic Activities (AA)—Perform one activity from the aerobic activities group each day. Participate in the activity at least 15 minutes.

Cool-down (CD)—Select three cool-down exercises each day from the suggested group or personal favorites. Exercises should stretch the upper body, the trunk, and the legs.

	Sunday	Monday	Tuesday	Wednesday	Thursday	Friday	Saturday
Week One Date:							
Week Two Date:							
Week Three Date:							
Week Four Date:							
Week Five Date:							
Week Six Date:							

Student Name: _____

What Is Your Resting Heart Rate?

When your fitness level improves, your resting heart rate may decrease as your heart becomes more efficient. To measure your resting heart rate, follow these steps.

1. A few minutes before going to sleep in the evening, lie down and relax for 2 or 3 minutes.

2. Use a wristwatch (or ask your parents to time you) and count your pulse for 6 seconds.

3. Add a zero to the end of the number to find your heart rate per minute.

4. Record your score on the chart.

Resting Heart Rate

	Sun	Mon	Tue	Wed	Thu	Fri	Sat
Week 1	___	___	___	___	___	___	___
Week 2	___	___	___	___	___	___	___
Week 3	___	___	___	___	___	___	___
Week 4	___	___	___	___	___	___	___
Week 5	___	___	___	___	___	___	___
Week 6	___	___	___	___	___	___	___

Target Heart Rate

If you are going to improve and maintain your aerobic fitness level, it is important that you move your heart rate into the target zone. The chart below shows when your heart rate is in the training zone:

If your resting heart rate is:	Target heart rate is:
Below 60	150
60–64	151
70–74	153
75–79	155
80–84	159
85–89	161
90 and over	163

Check your pulse rate 4 to 5 times a day during different types of activity. Record your heart rate below. Do you ever move your heart rate into the training zone during the day? How about during the entire week?

Monday _____ _____ _____ _____ _____

Tuesday _____ _____ _____ _____ _____

Wednesday _____ _____ _____ _____ _____

Thursday _____ _____ _____ _____ _____

Friday _____ _____ _____ _____ _____

Saturday _____ _____ _____ _____ _____

Sunday _____ _____ _____ _____ _____

VA 2.10

Your Activity and the Training Zone

Some activities are better than others for increasing your heart rate. On different days, participate in one of the activities listed below. After playing for exactly 5 minutes, stop and take your pulse rate. Record your score.

Activity	Heart Rate
Basketball	_____
Calisthenics	_____
Cycling	_____
Dance Aerobics	_____
Football	_____
Hockey	_____
Jogging	_____
Recess	_____
Rope Jumping	_____
Soccer	_____
Softball	_____
Walking	_____

Aerobic or Anaerobic Activity?

Some activities are best suited for improving aerobic capacity (with oxygen), while others primarily contribute to the anaerobic system (without oxygen). Both types of activities increase the breathing rate; however, anaerobic activities become so demanding they can only be done for a short time. In some cases, activities like basketball can contribute to both areas. Usually, anaerobic activities cannot be done longer than 2 minutes due to their demanding nature. As you participate in a number of activities, evaluate whether they are aerobic, anaerobic, or both.

Activity	Aerobic	Anaerobic	Both
Basketball	_____	_____	_____
Bowling	_____	_____	_____
Exercises	_____	_____	_____
Fitness Aerobics	_____	_____	_____
Football	_____	_____	_____
Gymnastics	_____	_____	_____
Hockey	_____	_____	_____
Jogging	_____	_____	_____
Rope Jumping	_____	_____	_____
Soccer	_____	_____	_____
Sprinting	_____	_____	_____
Swimming	_____	_____	_____
Walking	_____	_____	_____

Test Taking

One Mile Run/Walk or the PACER

◆ *Pace*
◆ *Run Correctly*

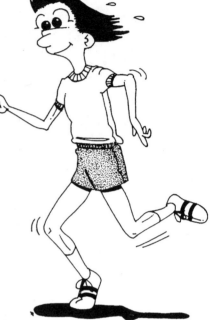

Curl-Up

◆ *Lift the Trunk*
◆ *Do It Correctly*

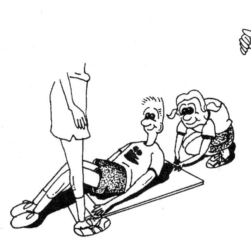

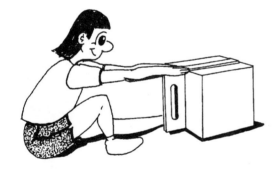

Sit-and-Reach

◆ *Stretch*

Push-Up

◆ *Keep Body Straight*
◆ *Correct Elbow Bend*
◆ *Hand Position*

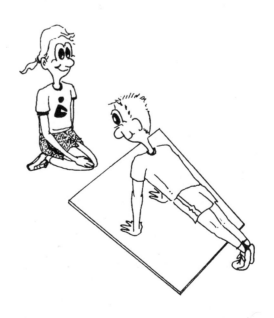

Pace, Don't Race!

To run a mile in your best time, you must learn to pace yourself. If you run 40 yards in the following times, you would have to continue that pace to run a mile in the time listed. Practice running 40 yards at different speeds to see which best suits your ability.

You must run 40 yards in:	To run a mile in:
8.2 seconds	6:00 minutes
9.5 seconds	7:00 minutes
10.9 seconds	8:00 minutes
12.3 seconds	9:00 minutes
13.6 seconds	10:00 minutes
15.0 seconds	11:00 minutes
16.4 seconds	12:00 minutes
17.7 seconds	13:00 minutes

Learning to Run

- *Head Up*

- *Chest Up*

- *Arm Swing (straight forward and back)*

- *Elbows Bent (90 degrees)*

- *Slight Forward Lean*

- *Foot and Leg Swing (straight forward and back)*

- *Longer Step Than Walking*

- *Whole Foot or Heel Hits Ground*

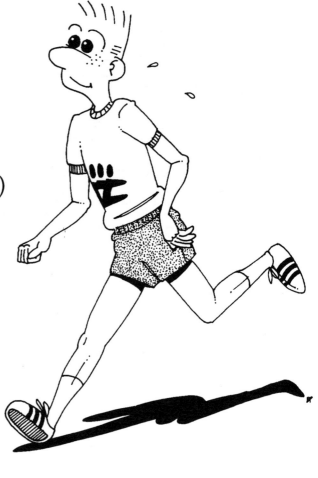

(Adapted from C. B. Corbin and R. Lindsey, *Fitness for Life*, 3rd ed. Glenview, IL: Scott, Foresman and Co., 1990.)

VA 2.15

FITNESSGRAM Body Composition Conversion Chart

BOYS*

Total MM	% FAT	Total MM	% FAT	Total MM	% FAT	Total MM	% FAT	Total MM	% FAT
1.0	1.7	16.0	12.8	31.0	23.8	46.0	34.8	61.0	45.8
1.5	2.1	16.5	13.1	31.5	24.2	46.5	35.2	61.5	46.2
2.0	2.5	17.0	13.5	32.0	24.5	47.0	35.5	62.0	46.6
2.5	2.8	17.5	13.9	32.5	24.9	47.5	35.9	62.5	46.9
3.0	3.2	18.0	14.2	33.0	25.3	48.0	36.3	63.0	47.3
3.5	3.6	18.5	14.6	33.5	25.6	48.5	36.6	63.5	47.7
4.0	3.9	19.0	15.0	34.0	26.0	49.0	37.0	64.0	48.0
4.5	4.3	19.5	15.3	34.5	26.4	49.5	37.4	64.5	48.4
5.0	4.7	20.0	15.7	35.0	26.7	50.0	37.8	65.0	48.8
5.5	5.0	20.5	16.1	35.5	27.1	50.5	38.1	65.5	49.1
6.0	5.4	21.0	16.4	36.0	27.5	51.0	38.5	66.0	49.5
6.5	5.8	21.5	16.8	36.5	27.8	51.5	38.9	66.5	49.9
7.0	6.1	22.0	17.2	37.0	28.2	52.0	39.2	67.0	50.2
7.5	6.5	22.5	17.5	37.5	28.6	52.5	39.6	67.5	50.6
8.0	6.9	23.0	17.9	38.0	28.9	53.0	40.0	68.0	51.0
8.5	7.2	23.5	18.3	38.5	29.3	53.5	40.3	68.5	51.3
9.0	7.6	24.0	18.6	39.0	29.7	54.0	40.7	69.0	51.7
9.5	8.0	24.5	19.0	39.5	30.0	54.5	41.1	69.5	52.1
10.0	8.4	25.0	19.4	40.0	30.4	55.0	41.4	70.0	52.5
10.5	8.7	25.5	19.7	40.5	30.8	55.5	41.8	70.5	52.8
11.0	9.1	26.0	20.1	41.0	31.1	56.0	42.2	71.0	53.2
11.5	9.5	26.5	20.5	41.5	31.5	56.5	42.5	71.5	53.6
12.0	9.8	27.0	20.8	42.0	31.9	57.0	42.9	72.0	53.9
12.5	10.2	27.5	21.2	42.5	32.2	57.5	43.3	72.5	54.3
13.0	10.6	28.0	21.6	43.0	32.6	58.0	43.6	73.0	54.7
13.5	10.9	28.5	21.9	43.5	33.0	58.5	44.0	73.5	55.0
14.0	11.3	29.0	22.3	44.0	33.3	59.0	44.4	74.0	55.4
14.5	11.7	29.5	22.7	44.5	33.7	59.5	44.7	74.5	55.8
15.0	12.0	30.0	23.1	45.0	34.1	60.0	45.1	75.0	56.1
15.5	12.4	30.5	23.4	45.5	34.4	60.5	45.5	75.5	56.5

* Use the chart to determine percent body fat for all boys ages 5 - 16+.

VA 2.16a

FITNESSGRAM Body Composition
Conversion Chart

GIRLS*

Total MM	% FAT	Total MM	% FAT	Total MM	% FAT	Total MM	% FAT	Total MM	% FAT
1.0	5.7	16.0	14.9	31.0	24.0	46.0	33.2	61.0	42.3
1.5	6.0	16.5	15.2	31.5	24.3	46.5	33.5	61.5	42.6
2.0	6.3	17.0	15.5	32.0	24.6	47.0	33.8	62.0	42.9
2.5	6.6	17.5	15.8	32.5	24.9	47.5	34.1	62.5	43.2
3.0	6.9	18.0	16.1	33.0	25.2	48.0	34.4	63.0	43.5
3.5	7.2	18.5	16.4	33.5	25.5	48.5	34.7	63.5	43.8
4.0	7.5	19.0	16.7	34.0	25.8	49.0	35.0	64.0	44.1
4.5	7.8	19.5	17.0	34.5	26.1	49.5	35.3	64.5	44.4
5.0	8.2	20.0	17.3	35.0	26.5	50.0	35.6	65.0	44.8
5.5	8.5	20.5	17.6	35.5	26.8	50.5	35.9	65.5	45.1
6.0	8.8	21.0	17.9	36.0	27.1	51.0	36.2	66.0	45.4
6.5	9.1	21.5	18.2	36.5	27.4	51.5	36.5	66.5	45.7
7.0	9.4	22.0	18.5	37.0	27.7	52.0	36.8	67.0	46.0
7.5	9.7	22.5	18.8	37.5	28.0	52.5	37.1	67.5	46.3
8.0	10.0	23.0	19.1	38.0	28.3	53.0	37.4	68.0	46.6
8.5	10.3	23.5	19.4	38.5	28.6	53.5	37.7	68.5	46.9
9.0	10.6	24.0	19.7	39.0	28.9	54.0	38.0	69.0	47.2
9.5	10.9	24.5	20.0	39.5	29.2	54.5	38.3	69.5	47.5
10.0	11.2	25.0	20.4	40.0	29.5	55.0	38.7	70.0	47.8
10.5	11.5	25.5	20.7	40.5	29.8	55.5	39.0	70.5	48.1
11.0	11.8	26.0	21.0	41.0	30.1	56.0	39.3	71.0	48.4
11.5	12.1	26.5	21.3	41.5	30.4	56.5	39.6	71.5	48.7
12.0	12.4	27.0	21.6	42.0	30.7	57.0	39.9	72.0	49.0
12.5	12.7	27.5	21.9	42.5	31.0	57.5	40.2	72.5	49.3
13.0	13.0	28.0	22.2	43.0	31.3	58.0	40.5	73.0	49.6
13.5	13.3	28.5	22.5	43.5	31.6	58.5	40.8	73.5	49.9
14.0	13.6	29.0	22.8	44.0	31.9	59.0	41.1	74.0	50.2
14.5	13.9	29.5	23.1	44.5	32.2	59.5	41.4	74.5	50.5
15.0	14.3	30.0	23.4	45.0	32.6	60.0	41.7	75.0	50.9
15.5	14.6	30.5	23.7	45.5	32.9	60.5	42.0	75.5	51.2

* Use the chart to determine percent body fat for all girls ages 5 - 16+.

VA 2.16b

Fitness Test
Warm-up and Cool-down

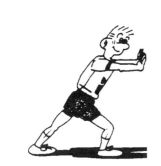

◆ *Calf Stretch*

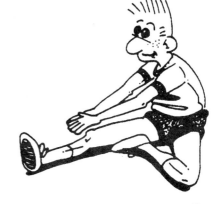

◆ *Sitting Toe-Touch*

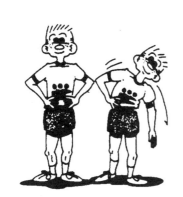

◆ *Side Bend*

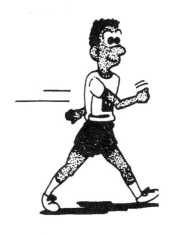

◆ *Walk or Slow Jog*

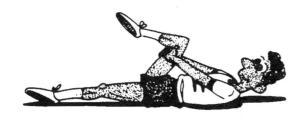

◆ *One-Leg Hug*

Reasons for Warm-up and Cool-down

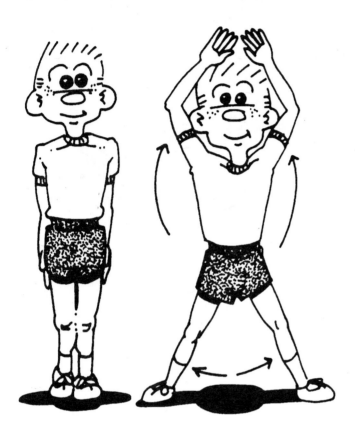

Warm-up

- ◆ *Prevent Injury*
- ◆ *Improve Performance*
- ◆ *Prevent Soreness*

Cool-down

- ◆ *Help Recovery*
- ◆ *Prevent Soreness*

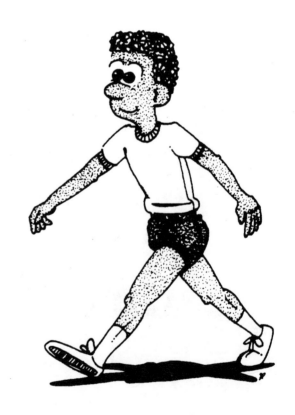

VA 2.18

Name _____ Date _____

♦ Fill out before taking the Prudential FITNESSGRAM Test.

♦ Circle the name of the test that you took. Write down your expected score for each test. You cannot be certain how you will do, give your best estimate.

♦ Darken the space in the boxes below. If your think you will score below the Healthy Fitness Zone, darken in the Needs Improvement area only. If you think you will score you will score in the Healthy Fitness Zone, darken into the shaded area. The farther you darken into the acceptable range the higher you think your score will be. For skinfold darken the "too low" area if you think you have too little body fat. Darken the "too high" area if you have too much body fat. Darken in the Healthy Fitness Zone if you think your body fat is in the healthy range.

	Estimated Score	**Estimated Fitness Range**

HEALTHY FITNESS ZONE

The PACER
One Mile Run/Walk
_____
Laps / Min. Sec.

Needs Improvement	Good	Better

Curl-ups
_____
Number

Needs Improvement	Good	Better

Trunk Lift
_____
Inches

Needs Improvement	Good	Better

Push-ups
Modified Pull-ups
Pull-ups
Flexed-Arm Hang
_____
Number / Seconds

Needs Improvement	Good	Better

Back-Saver
  Sit-and-reach
Shoulder Stretch
_____
Right P or F / Left P or F

Needs Improvement	Good	Better

Body Composition
(skinfolds)
_____
mm.

Needs Improvement	Good	Better

♦ After taking the Prudential FITNESSGRAM test, compare your estimate with your actual results.

Were you as fit as you thought you were? **YES   NO**

In what area were your estimates different from your actual test results?

VA 2.19

Feelings About Fitness Tests

◆ Read each of the statements about physical fitness tests.

◆ After reading the statements, circle one of the four responses.

◆ There are no correct or incorrect answers. Use the response that indicates how you feel about fitness tests.

◆ **DO NOT** put your name on this sheet.

	Never True For Me	Sometimes True For Me	Usually True For Me	Always True For Me
1. I enjoy taking fitness tests.	X	X	X	X
2. Taking fitness tests embarrasses me.	X	X	X	X
3. I am good at most fitness tests.	X	X	X	X
4. Most fitness test are fair.	X	X	X	X
5. I don't like to do fitness tests in front of friends.	X	X	X	X
6. Fitness tests make me sweat and mess up my hair so I don't like them.	X	X	X	X
7. I like to take fitness tests to see how well I can do.	X	X	X	X
8. I get nervous when I take fitness tests.	X	X	X	X
9. Most fitness tests give a good picture of true fitness.	X	X	X	X
10. Taking a fitness test seems like work.	X	X	X	X

List any other reasons you do or do not like to take fitness tests.

List some things that could be done to make fitness tests more fun or a better learning experience.

VA 2.20

My Personal Fitness Record

Name _____ Age _____ School _____ Grade _____

	Trial 1		Trial 2		Trial 3	
	Score	**HFZ**	**Score**	**HFZ**	**Score**	**HFZ**
Mile Run/Walk or the PACER	_____	_____	_____	_____	_____	_____
Triceps Skinfold	_____		_____		_____	
Calf Skinfold	_____		_____		_____	
Total Skinfold	_____	_____	_____	_____	_____	_____
Curl-up	_____	_____	_____	_____	_____	_____
Back-Saver Sit-and-Reach	_____	_____	_____	_____	_____	_____
Push-ups or Alternate Test	_____	_____	_____	_____	_____	_____
Trunk Lift	_____	_____	_____	_____	_____	_____
Other	_____	_____	_____	_____	_____	_____
Date of Testing	_____		_____		_____	

Note: HFZ indicates you have performed in the Healthy Fitness Zone.

I understand that my fitness record is personal. I do not have to share my results. My fitness record is important since it allows me to check my fitness level. If it is low, I will need to do more activity. If it is acceptable, I need to continue my current activity level. I know that I can ask my teacher for ideas for improving my fitness level.

A Brief Explanation...

Dear Parents,

This is a personal fitness record of your child. It is used to help students learn to monitor their fitness levels. Since it is a learning activity completed by your youngster, the results may not be entirely accurate.

The **test items** are designed to test health-related physical fitness. The purpose of each of the items is as follows:

One Mile Run/Walk or the PACER: Measures aerobic capacity, which is the best indicator of cardiovascular fitness. Cardio-vascular fitness will help prevent heart disease and obesity.

Skinfolds: Measures body composition, which reflects the amount of body fat. Excess body fat may cause health problems (diabetes or high blood pressure) and usually decreases skill performance.

Curl-ups: Measures abdominal strength and endurance, which is important for proper posture and prevention of lower back pain.

Sit-and-Reach: Measures the flexibility of the lower back and posterior thighs. This is important for the prevention of lower back pain.

Push-ups: Measures upper body strength and endurance, which is important for posture and skill performance.

Trunk Lift: Measures muscle fitness and flexibility of trunk, which is important for posture and back pain prevention.

The results are listed in two categories: the actual scores and an indication of whether the performance was in the Healthy Fitness Zone. It is reasonable to expect your child to score in the Healthy Fitness Zone since he or she is not compared to other youngsters, but to standards that indicate good health.

VA 3.1

The Prudential FITNESSGRAM
Class Score Sheet

Teacher _____

Class _____

Page Number _____

Grade _____

Test Date _____

ID#	Name	Birth Date	Sex	Height	Weight	Aerobic Capacity	Curl-up	Upper Body	Trunk Lift	Flexibility L/R	Skinfolds Triceps	Calf

VA 3.2

Measuring Body Composition

Location of Body Fat

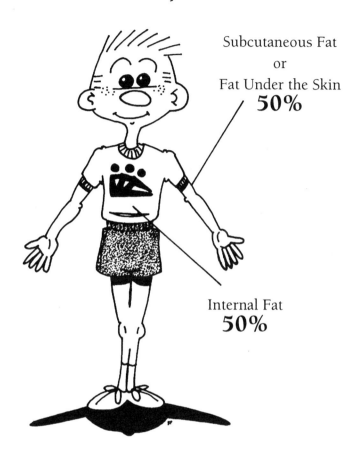

Subcutaneous Fat
or
Fat Under the Skin
50%

Internal Fat
50%

Skinfold Measuring

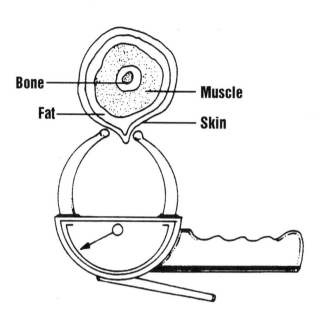

Bone

Fat

Muscle

Skin

Too Much Fat

◆ Increased chance of disease (heart disease, diabetes)
◆ Detracts from optimal appearance
◆ May reduce performance efficiency

Too Little Fat

◆ Causes health problems
   (fat needed to use vitamins)
◆ Anorexia nervosa can be fatal
◆ Bulimia and anorexia can result in bad teeth, stomach problems
◆ Detracts from optimal appearance

Aerobic Capacity—One Mile Run/Walk

To test your aerobic capacity, use the following steps:

1. Find a friend to time you during the mile run/walk.

2. Give your scorecard to your friend to record your score when you are finished.

3. If you are timing someone, make a mark on the scorecard each time your partner completes a lap.

4. Pace yourself. Remember to pace, not race. If you run too fast in the early part of the race, you will find it difficult to complete the run.

5. You may walk if you have to; however, the goal is to finish the mile in the least amount of time. Try to use a steady jogging pace.

6. Enjoy yourself—the results are for you and give an indication of your aerobic capacity.

One Mile Run/Walk Using 220-Yard Track

Lap #1 _____   Lap #5 _____

Lap #2 _____   Lap #6 _____

Lap #3 _____   Lap #7 _____

Lap #4 _____   Lap #8 _____

Mile Run/Walk Time _____

VA 3.4

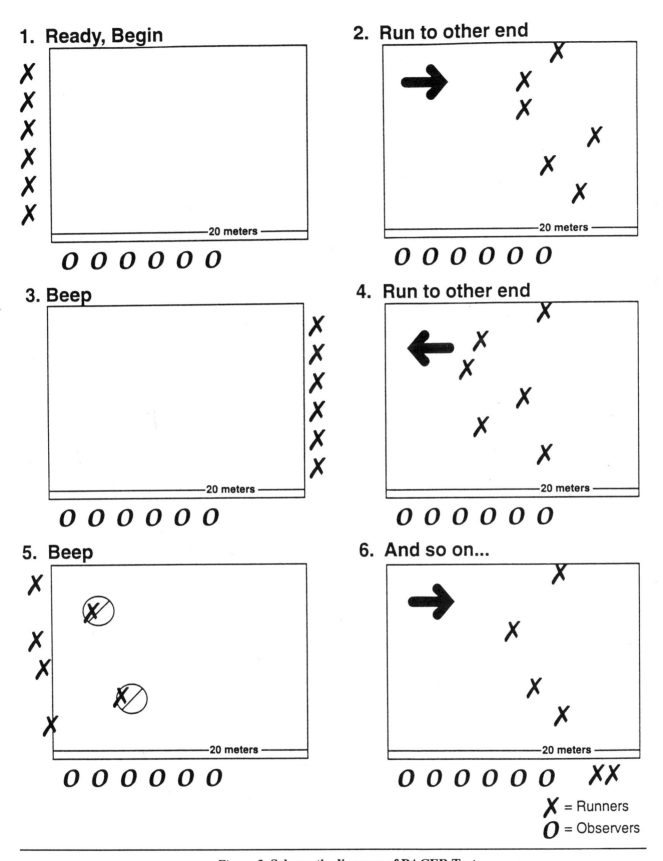

1. **Ready, Begin**

2. **Run to other end**

3. **Beep**

4. **Run to other end**

5. **Beep**

6. **And so on...**

20 meters

X = Runners
O = Observers

Figure 2. **Schematic diagram of PACER Test.**

VA 3.5

Body Composition— Skinfold Measurements

Triceps

1. Find a friend to measure you.

2. Your friend will measure your skinfold thickness, and you will record the results on your card.

3. Measure the right triceps skinfold first. Place one end of the string on the tip of the shoulder and the other on the tip of the elbow. Fold the string in half and place both ends in one hand. Place the ends of the folded string on the shoulder tip. The folded end is placed on the triceps muscle. Mark this spot with a marking pencil.

4. Grasp the skinfold slightly above the mark and measure the thickness of the skinfold on the mark. Grasp the skinfold firmly and lift it away from the muscle. Do not pinch too hard.

5. Read the skinfold to the nearest millimeter.

6. Make three measurements and record the middle score if the results are different on the measurements.

7. Change roles with your partner. When finished, move on to the calf measurement.

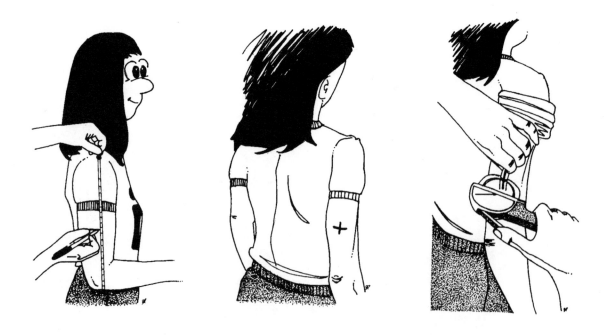

VA 3.6

Body Composition— Skinfold Measurements

Calf

1. Your friend will measure your calf skinfold thickness, and you will record the results on your card.

2. Place your right foot on the elevated surface so the knee is bent at a 90 degree angle as shown below. Mark the measurement spot on the inside and largest part of the calf.

3. Grasp the skinfold slightly above the mark and measure the thickness of the skinfold on the mark as shown below. Grasp the skinfold firmly and lift it away from the muscle. Do not pinch too hard.

4. Read the skinfold to the nearest millimeter.

5. Make three measurements and record the middle score if the results are different on each of the measurements.

6. Change roles with your partner.

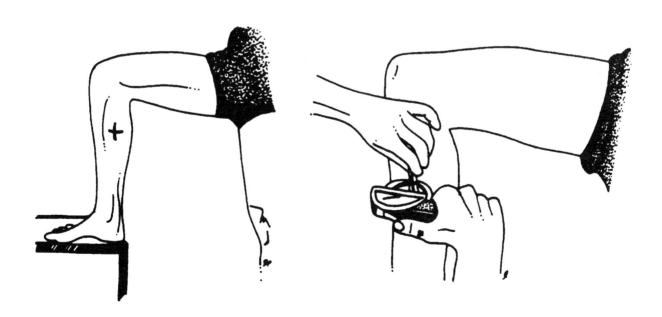

Flexibility—Back-Saver Sit-and-Reach

1. Find a friend to help you measure and record your score.

2. Take off your shoes.

3. Sit at the sit-and-reach box with one leg straight and the same foot against the box. Bend the other leg with the sole of the foot flat on the floor. Place your hands on top of each other, and place them on top of the box as shown below.

4. Your partner should place his or her hands on your knee to keep it from bending.

5. Reach forward with both hands along the measuring scale 4 times and hold the position of your best reach on the fourth trial.

6. You must hold your best reach for at least 1 second. Do not count the score if it is the result of bouncing forward without holding the reach position.

7. The score is measured to the nearest half-inch.

8. Repeat with the other leg.

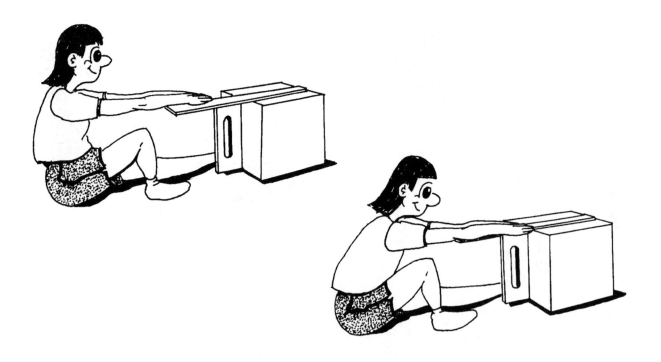

VA 3.8

Abdominal Fitness—Curl-up Test

1. Find two friends to help you do the test and record your results.

2. Lie on the mat with your knees bent at a 140 degree angle and the soles of the feet flat on the floor.

3. The arms are straight at the sides with palms open and against the mat.

4. One partner places the measuring strip under the knees on the mat so the edge of the strip is at the fingertips. The partner then assumes a position with the hands under the head.

5. The other partner stands on the measuring strip, one foot on either side.

6. A curl-up is counted when the fingers touch the opposite side of the measuring strip.

7. When your partner says "go," see how many curl-ups you can do.

8. Do the curl-ups on the cadence (one every 3 seconds).

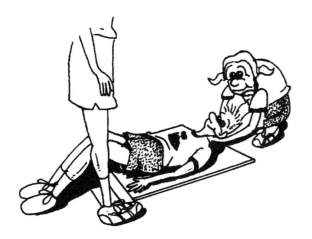

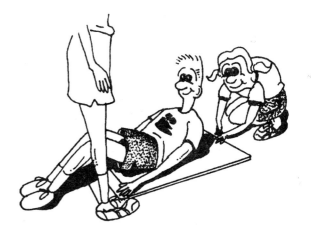

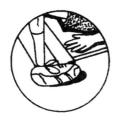 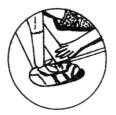

Upper-Body Fitness—Push-ups

1. Find a friend to help you with the tests and record your results.

2. Lie face down on the floor. Place your hands under your shoulders with your fingers spread.

3. Keep your body and legs straight with your feet slightly apart and toes tucked under.

4. Push up off the mat until your arms are straight. Your back should be kept in a straight line from head to toe.

5. Lower your body until the arms are bent at 90 degrees. The upper part of the arm will be parallel to the floor.

6. Repeat by moving up on "up" and down on "down." Do one push up every 3 seconds (20 per minute).

7. Your partner will count for you. Repeat until you cannot continue.

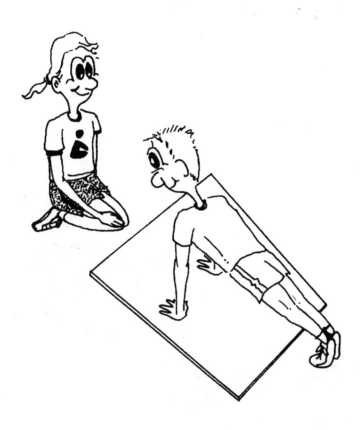

Trunk Lift

1. Find a friend to help you with the test and record your results.

2. Lie on a mat face down. Point your toes away from your body. Place your hands under your thighs.

3. Lift your upper body (trunk) off the floor slowly. Do not jerk when lifting off the floor.

4. Lift as high as you can up to 12 inches. Do not lift higher than 12 inches.

5. Your partner will measure the distance you lift your chin off the mat with a flexible rule and will record your score.

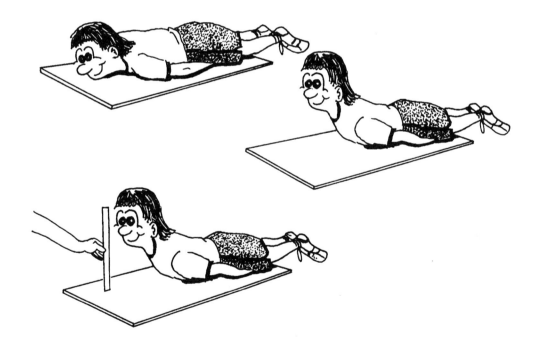

Fitness Testing Homework

Dear Parent:

          is most interested in the physical fitness of your child. We are currently involved in preparing students for the upcoming fitness tests. Physical education and fitness will improve when homework is completed by your child. I would like to ask you to help your child prepare for the upcoming mile run/walk by participating with your child in these activities.

The following are activities that will help your child improve his/her performance. These activities have been selected as favorites by your child. Please write in the amount of time you and your child participated in the activities.

Family Participation

Sunday	_____	_____	_____
Monday	_____	_____	_____
Tuesday	_____	_____	_____
Wednesday	_____	_____	_____
Thursday	_____	_____	_____
Friday	_____	_____	_____
Saturday	_____	_____	_____

Stairway to Lifetime Fitness

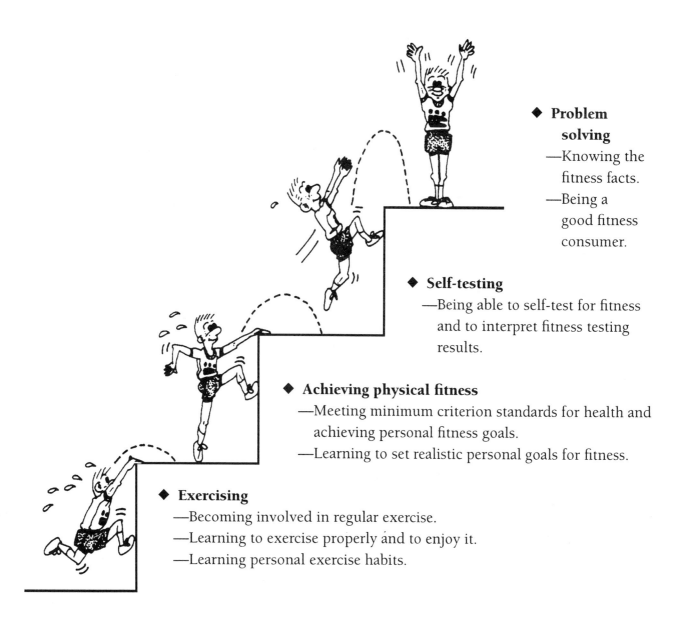

◆ **Problem solving**
  —Knowing the fitness facts.
  —Being a good fitness consumer.

◆ **Self-testing**
  —Being able to self-test for fitness and to interpret fitness testing results.

◆ **Achieving physical fitness**
  —Meeting minimum criterion standards for health and achieving personal fitness goals.
  —Learning to set realistic personal goals for fitness.

◆ **Exercising**
  —Becoming involved in regular exercise.
  —Learning to exercise properly and to enjoy it.
  —Learning personal exercise habits.

CALENDAR

Sunday	Monday	Tuesday	Wednesday	Thursday	Friday	Saturday

VA 4.2

What Do Exercises Do for Your Body?

List below some of the exercises you have learned in class. Then evaluate what they do for your body. Place a mark in the column that you think describes what the exercise does for you.

Exercise	Aerobic Capacity	Flexibility	Muscular Strength
_____	_____	_____	_____
_____	_____	_____	_____
_____	_____	_____	_____
_____	_____	_____	_____
_____	_____	_____	_____
_____	_____	_____	_____
_____	_____	_____	_____
_____	_____	_____	_____
_____	_____	_____	_____
_____	_____	_____	_____
_____	_____	_____	_____
_____	_____	_____	_____
_____	_____	_____	_____
_____	_____	_____	_____

Work Hard, Keep Fit

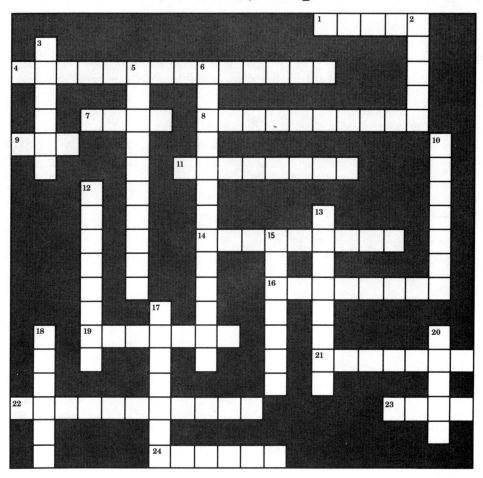

ACROSS CLUES

1. The "Bulb" muscle in your arms when you "make a muscle."
4. _____ fitness refers to the fitness of the heart, body organ.
7. A well-balanced diet provides the _____ for physical activity.
8. Experts believe people are _____ due to the lack of activity rather than because they eat too much.
9. P.E. is _____.
11. Bones become _____ in response to regular exercise.
14. Sit-ups or curl-ups develop your_____ muscles.
16. If you want to improve your fitness, you must do regular _____.
19. _____ activities include jogging, swimming, biking, walking, and dancing.
21. _____ are the body tissues that work when you exercise.
22. Endurance, _____, body composition and strength are the elements of health-related fitness.
23. It takes a lot of hard _____ to stay in good physical condition.
24. Skip, hop, ____, leap, slide, run, jump, and walk are the eight basic locomotor movements.

DOWN CLUES

2. _____ is a quick change of direction.
3. _____ is essential before participating in strenuous activities.
5. Sweating occurs when the body is _____ and helps to maintain a constant body temperature.
6. Good _____ is essential in any team situation.
10. In _____ stunts, the center of weight. must be positioned over the base of support.
12. In terms of _____ exertion, 10 minutes of rope jumping is equal to 30 minutes of jogging.
13. Activities you can do throughout most of your life are called _____ sports.
15. _____ means extreme fatness.
17. _____ is one good way to increase aerobic endurance.
18. To maintain good _____, eat a balanced diet and follow regular program of exercise.
20. The _____ is a muscle that works like a pump.

VA 4.4a

Work Hard, Keep Fit

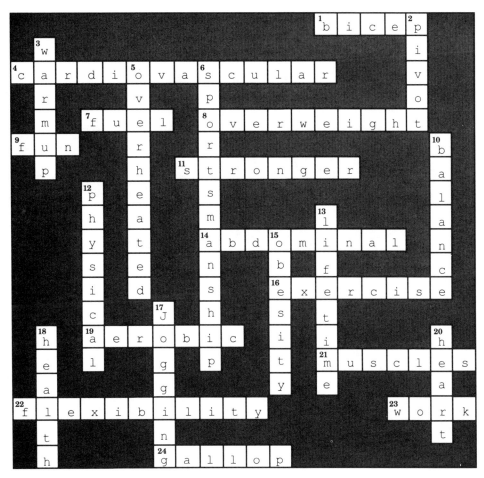

ACROSS CLUES

1. The "Bulb" muscle in your arms when you "make a muscle."
4. _____ fitness refers to the fitness of the heart, body organ.
7. A well-balanced diet provides the _____ for physical activity.
8. Experts believe people are _____ due to the lack of activity rather than because they eat too much.
9. P.E. is _____.
11. Bones become _____ in response to regular exercise.
14. Sit-ups or curl-ups develop your_____ muscles.
16. If you want to improve your fitness, you must do regular _____.
19. _____ activities include jogging, swimming, biking, walking, and dancing.
21. _____ are the body tissues that work when you exercise.
22. Endurance, _____, body composition and strength are the elements of health-related fitness.
23. It takes a lot of hard _____ to stay in good physical condition.
24. Skip, hop, ____, leap, slide, run, jump, and walk are the eight basic locomotor movements.

DOWN CLUES

2. _____ is a quick change of direction.
3. _____ is essential before participating in strenuous activities.
5. Sweating occurs when the body is _____ and helps to maintain a constant body temperature.
6. Good _____ is essential in any team situation.
10. In _____ stunts, the center of weight must be positioned over the base of support.
12. In terms of _____ exertion, 10 minutes of rope jumping is equal to 30 minutes of jogging.
13. Activities you can do throughout most of your life are called _____ sports.
15. _____ means extreme fatness.
17. _____ is one good way to increase aerobic endurance.
18. To maintain good _____, eat a balanced diet and follow regular program of exercise.
20. The _____ is a muscle that works like a pump.

GET FIT!!

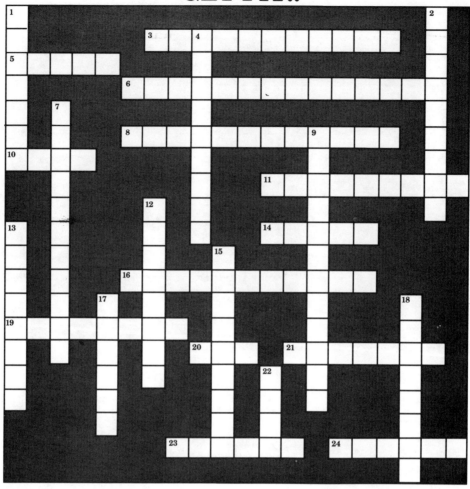

Across Clues

3. The principle of _____ states that you must do specific exercises to build specific parts of fitness.
5. You do not need a lot of _____ to develop physical fitness.
6. _____refers to the heart and blood vessels.
8. _____ is the ability to use your senses together with your body parts.
10. There is no _____ way to become physically fit.
11. _____ refers to how hard you must work to improve your level of fitness.
14. _____ is the movement of blood through your arteries caused by the heart beating.
16. Increasing the overload amounts of exercise gradually, refers to the principle of _____.
19. To be beneficial, the _____ of each bout of exercise must be at least 15 - 20 minutes.
20. P.E. is _____!
21. _____ means with oxygen.
23. The blood carries_____ to the muscles.
24. _____-related fitness helps you resist conditions caused by lack of exercise.

Down Clues

1. Obesity is one risk factor that leads to heart _____.
2. Your _____ _____ is the number of times the heart beats per minute.
4. Cardiovascular _____ (aerobic capicity) is the ability to exercise the entire body for long periods of time.
7. The _____ system is made up of the lungs and air passages.
9. _____ _____ includes physical, mental, social, and emotional fitness.
12. The priniciple of _____ refers to increasing the amount of exercise you do each time you exercise.
13. It is important to _____ - _____ (continue moving) following strenuous exercise.
15. _____ deals with how often you must exercise to improve your physical fitness.
17. Active people have a reduced rate of heart _____.
18. A _____measures your body fatness.
22. We _____P.E.

GET FIT!!

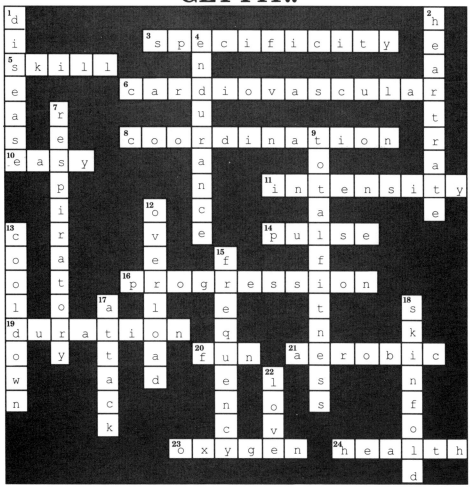

Across Clues

3. The principle of _____ states that you must do specific exercises to build specific parts of fitness.
5. You do not need a lot of _____ to develop physical fitness.
6. _____ refers to the heart and blood vessels.
8. _____ is the ability to use your senses together with your body parts.
10. There is no _____ way to become physically fit.
11. _____ refers to how hard you must work to improve your level of fitness.
14. _____ is the movement of blood through your arteries caused by the heart beating.
16. Increasing the overload amounts of exercise gradually, refers to the principle of _____.
19. To be beneficial, the _____ of each bout of exercise must be at least 15 - 20 minutes.
20. P.E. is _____!
21. _____ means with oxygen.
23. The blood carries_____ to the muscles.
24. _____-related fitness helps you resist conditions caused by lack of exercise.

Down Clues

1. Obesity is one risk factor that leads to heart _____.
2. Your _____ _____ is the number of times the heart beats per minute.
4. Cardiovascular _____ (aerobic capicity) is the ability to exercise the entire body for long periods of time.
7. The _____ system is made up of the lungs and air passages.
9. _____ _____ includes physical, mental, social, and emotional fitness.
12. The priniciple of _____ refers to increasing the amount of exercise you do each time you exercise.
13. It is important to _____ - _____ (continue moving) following strenuous exercise.
15. _____ deals with how often you must exercise to improve your physical fitness.
17. Active people have a reduced rate of heart _____.
18. A _____measures your body fatness.
22. We _____P.E.

VA 4.5b

Burning Calories Through Exercise*

You can burn calories by exercising. This chart will help you determine which types of exercise are more demanding. If you want to lose body fat, it is a good idåea to pick those activities which burn more calories.

Activity	Weight:	60 lbs	80 lbs	100 lbs
		Calories Used Per Hour		
Backpacking		226	267	307
Basketball		165	195	225
Bicycling		116	137	157
Bowling		115	136	155
Dance (Aerobic)		231	273	315
Calisthenics		171	202	232
Football		165	195	225
Hiking		165	195	225
Jogging		358	423	487
Rope Jumping		385	455	525
Running		495	585	625
Skating		193	228	262
Soccer		297	351	405
Softball		160	186	217
Swimming (slow)		176	208	240
Swimming (fast)		347	410	472
Volleyball		193	228	262
Walking		175	207	204

*(Adapted from C. B. Corbin and R. Lindsey, *Fitness for Life*, 3rd ed. Glenview, IL: Scott, Foresman and Co., 1990.)

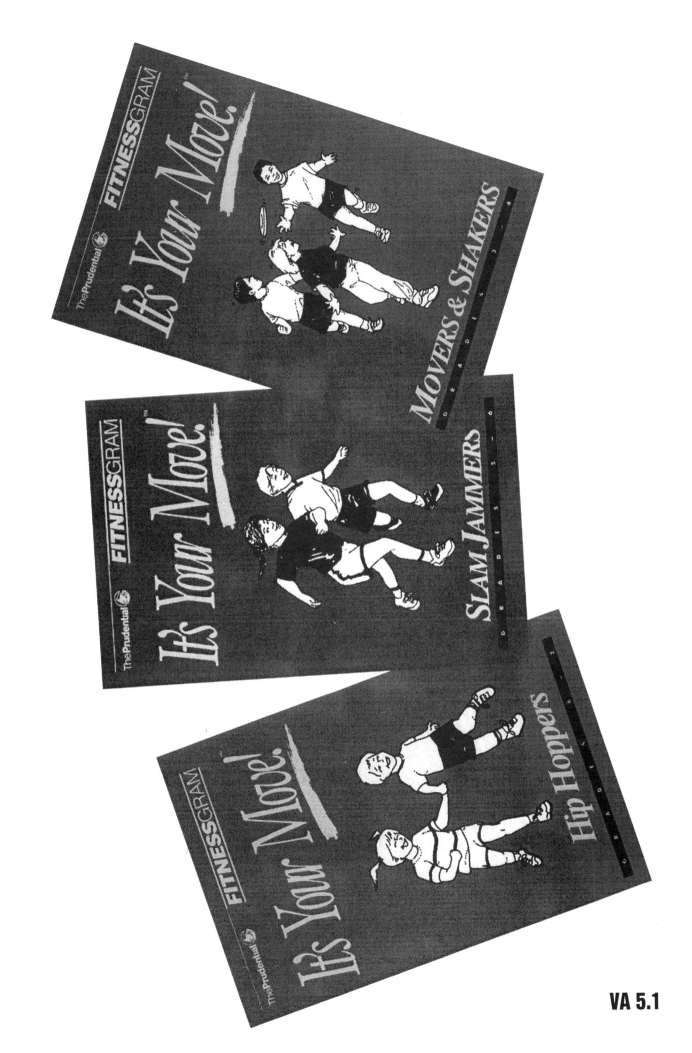

VA 5.1

Student/Adult Agreement

Before you start being a *Slam Jammer*, read and fill in this page with your helping adult.

I, _____, agree to take part in at least two activities from

each group in the booklet. When I have completed an activity I will tell my helping adult and

give them my booklet to initial. I understand that it is my job to keep up with my booklet.

_____

Child's Signature   Date

I, _____, understand that after my child completes

any activity in this booklet I must initial the appropriate box in the tracking chart at the bottom

of each page. I will also have my child initial the appropriate box.

_____

Helping Adult's Signature   Date

VA 5.2

Knowing about Fitness
Fourth Grade

You must finish at least two of the activities in this section before you give your booklet to your teacher. This part will help you understand more about fitness and health.

1. On a piece of paper, write the name of two exercises that work the following body parts.

Arms   Shoulders
Abdomen (stomach)   Back
Legs

2. Draw or paint your picture doing your favorite activity and show it to your parent or helping adult.

3. Make a list of ten foods that don't have a lot of fat. Write a one or two page report explaining why these foods are good for you to eat.

Date		
Activity Number		
Adult's Initials		

For each completed activity, enter the date, the activity number and the Adult's initials in the spaces provided.

The Active Days Chart is filled in and the *It's Your Move!* project was successfully completed.

_____
Child's Signature

_____
Adult's Signature

Date

Way To Go!

KEEP UP THE ACTIVITY!

Give this booklet to your teacher so you can put your star on the *Mover and Shaker* poster at school.

Group 2
Activities to do by Yourself

Do at least two of the following activities for 15 minutes or more. These activities should be fun for you and can be done all by yourself.

1. Ride your bike or go roller-skating.

2. Walk quickly to school, the bus stop, the shopping center or a friend's home.

3. Jog or go for a hike.

4. Make up a fitness routine which includes exercises and rope jumping or running in place. Exercise using your routine.

5. Play frisbee golf.

6. Shoot baskets.

7. Dribble a soccer ball and practice shooting on goal.

8. Pitch a baseball against a wall.

9. Swim and play at the pool. Make certain that a lifeguard is on duty.

10. Take your pet for a walk.

11. Jump rope.

 SAFETY ALERT Always get permission before doing any of these activities.

Date				
Activity Number				
Adult's Initials				

For each completed activity, enter the date, the activity number and the Adult's initials in the spaces provided.

Group 3
Activities with Friends

Take part in these or activities like these with friends for at least 15 minutes. Do at least two activities.

1. Play a game that takes 2-4 friends such as tennis, two-on-two basketball, two person volleyball, four square or hopscotch.

2. Ride bikes with your friends.

3. Find a different way to walk to school or the bus stop and back home with your friends. Make the walk longer each time, until it takes 15 minutes to get home. Make certain that your parent or helping adult knows what way you will walk and what time you will be home.

4. Find a friend to help you test your fitness. Measure yourself using the *FITNESSGRAM* test.

5. Go for a hike, a walk or a jog with a friend.

6. Try an activity you haven't done before such as: swimming, exercises, roller skating, ice skating or make-up a new game.

SAFETY ALERT Always get permission before doing any of these activities.

Date						
Activity Number						
Adult's Initials						

For each completed activity, enter the date, the activity number and the Adult's initials in the spaces provided.

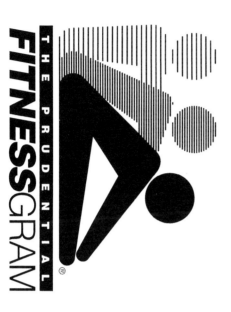

In recognition of outstanding achievement
in health and fitness

The Prudential **FITNESSGRAM** program
presents this certificate to:

Date

Instructor

Principal

VA 5.5

The Prudential FITNESSGRAM "Fit for Life" program is designed to promote exercise as an important part of each day. It provides a means of monitoring physical activity over an 8- to 10-week period, and makes incentives available to individuals who record good exercise habits. Children, youth and adults are encouraged to exercise together. Here's what to do:

1 Try to get some kind of physical activity at least three or four days each week.

2 Consult the table below to determine how many points you have earned each day and record them on the activity log. Be proud of each point! Points may be earned from one or several activities. You should try to earn at least 2 points each day.

3 Earn as many points each week as you'd like. However, only the maximum number of points per week listed below will count toward successful completion.

4 Try to accumulate the total goal for your age group (see below) in an 8 week period. You may increase the time to 10 weeks if you are sick or injured.

5 Once you reach your point goal, you will receive a colorful 8"x10" certificate suitable for framing. Sign your completed activity log and send it to **Fit for Life, The Prudential FITNESSGRAM, 12330 Preston Rd., Dallas, TX 75230.**

Activity	Time	Points
Badminton	15 minutes	1
Basketball	20 minutes	2
Calisthenics	15 minutes	1
Cross Country Skiing	10 minutes	2
Cycling	15 minutes	1
Dance (Aerobics)	20 minutes	2
Dance (Tap, Ballet, Modern)	30 minutes	2
Field Hockey	20 minutes	2
Gymnastics	30 minutes	2
Ice Hockey/Field Hockey	20 minutes	2
Jogging/Running	10 minutes	2
Lacrosse	20 minutes	2
Martial Arts	20 minutes	1
Racquetball/Handball/Squash	20 minutes	2
Rope Jumping (Individual)	10 minutes	2
Skating (Ice/Roller)	15 minutes	1
Soccer	20 minutes	2
Swimming (Laps)	10 minutes	2
Tennis	15 minutes	1
Volleyball	30 minutes	2
Walking	15 minutes	2
Weight Training	15 minutes	1
Wrestling (Competitive)	20 minutes	2

Some activities will be more vigorous than others. Certain activities develop strength and flexibility, while others develop aerobic endurance. Point values are intended only for use in recording your activity.

Age	Total Points Needed	Maximum Points Per Week
5-8	80	10
9-12	120	15
13-17	160	20
17+	192	24

THE PRUDENTIAL FITNESSGRAM®

FIT FOR LIFE
ACTIVITY LOG

WEEK 1
Sun	Mon	Tues	Wed	Thurs	Fri	Sat

WEEK 2

WEEK 3

WEEK 4

WEEK 5

WEEK 6

WEEK 7

WEEK 8

WEEK 9

WEEK 10

Total Points Earned _____ Signature _____

Cooperating Agencies

The Cooper Institute for Aerobics Research is a non-profit research and education center dedicated to advancing the understanding of the relationship between living habits and health and to providing leadership in implementing these concepts to enhance the physical and emotional well-being of the individual.

The Prudential, America's largest insurance company, is committed to a wide range of programs designed to help people achieve and maintain good health throughout their lives.

Fitness Contract

I, _____, agree to:

When I complete the requirements listed above, I will receive The Prudential FITNESSGRAM honor award.

_____   _____
Student's Signature   Date

I agree that the student named above will receive The Prudential FITNESSGRAM honor award for completing the requirements named above.

_____   _____
Teacher's Signature   Date

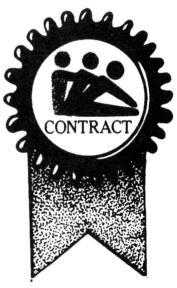

Exercise and Fitness Log

Name_____ Year _____–_____

Check one or both:
☐ **The PACER**
☐ **One Mile Run/Walk**

	Needs Improvement	Healthy Fitness Zone	Score
Date 1 _____			_____
Date 2 _____			_____
Date 3 _____			_____
Date 4 _____			_____

Body Composition

	Needs Improvement	Healthy Fitness Zone	Score
Date 1 _____			_____
Date 2 _____			_____
Date 3 _____			_____
Date 4 _____			_____

Curl-ups

	Needs Improvement	Healthy Fitness Zone	Score
Date 1 _____			_____
Date 2 _____			_____
Date 3 _____			_____
Date 4 _____			_____

VA 5.8a

Check one or more:
Back-Saver
Sit-and-Reach
Shoulder Stretch

	Needs Improvement	Healthy Fitness Zone	Score
Date 1 _____			_____
Date 2 _____			_____
Date 3 _____			_____
Date 4 _____			_____

Check one or more:
Push-ups
Pull-ups
Flexed-Arm Hang
Modified Pull-ups

	Needs Improvement	Healthy Fitness Zone	Score
Date 1 _____			_____
Date 2 _____			_____
Date 3 _____			_____
Date 4 _____			_____

Trunk Lift	Needs Improvement	Healthy Fitness Zone	Score
Date 1 _____			_____
Date 2 _____			_____
Date 3 _____			_____
Date 4 _____			_____

VA 5.8b

PHYSICAL ACTIVITY READINESS QUESTIONNAIRE
(PAR-Q)
A Self-Administered Questionnaire for Adults

PAR-Q is designed to help you help yourself. Many health benefits are associated with regular exercise, and the completion of PAR-Q is a sensible first step to take if you are planning to increase the amount of physical activity in your life.

For most people, physical activity should not pose any problem or hazard. PAR-Q has been designed to identify the small number of adults for whom physical activity might be inappropriate or those who should have medical advice concerning the type of activity most suitable for them.

Common sense is your best guide in answering these few questions. Please read them carefully and check ☑ YES or NO opposite the question if it applies to you.

YES   NO

☐   ☐   1. Has you doctor ever said you have heart trouble?

☐   ☐   2. Do you frequently have pains in your heart and chest?

☐   ☐   3. Do you often feel faint or have spells of severe dizziness?

☐   ☐   4. Has a doctor ever said your blood pressure was too high?

☐   ☐   5. Has you doctor ever told you that you have a bone or joint problem such has arthritis that has been aggravated by exercise, or might be made worse with exercise?

☐   ☐   6. Is there a good physical reason not mentioned here why you should not follow an activity program even if you wanted to?

☐   ☐   7. Are you over age 65 and not accustomed to vigorous exercise?

If You Answered ➡

YES to one or more questions

If you have not recently done so, consult with your personal physician by telephone or in person BEFORE increasing your physical activity and / or taking a fitness test. Tell him what questions you answered YES on PAR-Q, or show him your copy.

PROGRAMS

After medical evaluation, seek advice from your physician as to your suitability for:
+ unrestricted physical activity starting off easily and progressing gradually.
+ restricted or supervised activity to meet your specific needs, at least on an initial basis. Check in your community for special programs or services.

NO to all questions

If you answered PAR-Q accurately, you have reasonable assurance of your present suitability for:
+ *A Graduated Exercise Program* - A gradual increase in proper exercise promotes good fitness development while minimizing or eliminating discomfort.
+ *A Fitness Appraisal* - A simple tests of fitness (such as the Canadian Home Fitness Test) may be undertaken if you so desire.

POSTPONE

If you have a temporary minor illness, such as a common cold.

Developed by the British Columbia Ministry of Health.
Modified and used with the permission of the British Columbia Ministry of Health.

VA 6.1

Dear

We would like to invite you to attend a Prudential FITNESSGRAM Family Fitness Night. The purpose of the evening will be to acquaint you with The Prudential FITNESSGRAM program, which is a new and motivating approach to youth fitness. The Prudential FITNESSGRAM program uses a new recognition system that allows **all** youngsters to improve their fitness and be recognized.

Activities for the evening will include an opportunity to evaluate the fitness level of your child as well as your own personal fitness level. In addition, we will interpret the results of the testing and offer ideas for improving fitness at home.

It should be an exciting evening. I look forward to meeting you. Plan on being at the school by

Thanks for your help and support.

Sincerely,

Physical Education Instructor

Date:

Contact Person:

Contact Phone Number:

                    will be hosting a special night for students and parents for the purpose of introducing a new youth fitness program. The Prudential FITNESSGRAM fitness program is a new and motivating approach being implemented to improve fitness levels of school children. The Prudential FITNESSGRAM program uses a new recognition system that allows all youngsters to improve their fitness status and be recognized.

Parents will have the opportunity to evaluate the fitness levels of their children and learn how to interpret the results. Activities for improving fitness levels at home will be shared with participants.

It should be an evening filled with action and excitement. When parents and children evaluate each other, the result is always enjoyable and educational. The program will begin promptly at

Thanks for your help and support.

VA 6.3

Family-in-Training Profile

Answer the questions below to determine your family's attitude about nutrition, exercise, health, and fun...important elements in a successful fitness program.

(Check the best response for each of the questions below.)

	Yes	No
1. Do all members of your family exercise at least 3 times each week?	___	___
2. Are all members of your family as physically fit as they should be?	___	___
3. Are all members of your family at their best weight (not too fat or too thin)?	___	___
4. Do all members of your family eat a good breakfast each day?	___	___
5. Do all members of your family eat three regular meals each day?	___	___
6. Do all members of your family moderate their snacking?	___	___
7. Have all members of your family had a thorough physical examination in the last 2 years?	___	___
8. Do all members of your family understand the importance of having a release for stress?	___	___
9. Is your family free of smokers?	___	___
10. Does your family have a time each day to be together and talk (other than meal time)?	___	___
11. Is there at least one activity that all members of your family enjoy together?	___	___
12. Is your family involved in one away-from-home family activity at least once a week?	___	___

Scoring

1. Family exercise score—How many "yes" answers did your family have for the first three questions? _____

2. Family nutrition score—How many "yes" answers did your family have for questions 4, 5, and 6? _____

3. Family health score—How many "yes" answers did your family have for questions 7, 8, and 8? _____

4. Family fun score—How many "yes" answers did your family have for questions 10, 11, and 12? _____

Ratings

A score of 3 on any of the categories gives your family a good rating. Keep up the good work!

A score of 2 on any of the scores is "fair" but could be better. See where your family could improve.

A score of 0 to 1 on any of the scores means your family should make some changes. Improvement is important. Work together to make positive changes.

(Developed by C. B. Corbin and R. Pangrazi for the "Family in Training Program." Used with permission of Nabisco.)

Learning What Exercises Do for the Body

Exercises are usually classified according to their contribution to the development of the body. The following exercises have been taught to your child. Ask them (or let them) to show you how to perform each one and see if they know what area of the body is developed.

General Body Activities—Aerobic Fitness:
> Rope jumping, running in place, tortoise and hare, and the PACER

Arm–Shoulder Girdle Exercises:
> Crab walk, crab kick, and rope climbing

Leg Exercises:
> Step-ups, straddle bench jumps, and agility run

Arm and Shoulder Exercises:
> Flexed-arm hang, push-ups, lying arm circles

Abdominal Exercises:
> Curl-ups, alternate toe touching

Flexibility Exercises:
> Bend-and-stretch, calf stretch, and trunk twist

Aerobic and Partner Resistance Exercises

Aerobic activity can involve a wide variety of movements, including rope jumping, jogging, fast walking, and animal walks. Alternate 1 minute of an aerobic activity with 1 minute of partner resistance exercises. The total routine should include a minimum of 5 minutes of aerobic exercise and 5 minutes of partner resistance activity.

Partner Resistance Exercises

Arm Curl-up—Exerciser keeps the upper arms against the sides with the forearms and palms forward. Partner puts fists in exerciser's palms. Exerciser attempts to curl the forearms upward to the shoulders. To develop the opposite set of muscles, partners reverse hand positions. Palms begin at shoulder level and push down in opposite direction.

Shoulder Flexion—Exerciser extends the arms and places the hands, palms down, on partner's shoulders. Exerciser attempts to push partner into the floor. Partner may slowly lower himself to allow the exerciser movement through the range of motion.

Fist Pull-Apart—Exerciser places the fists together in front of the body at shoulder level. Exerciser attempts to pull the hands apart while partner forces them together with pressure on the elbows. As a variation, with fists apart, the exerciser tries to push them together. Partner applies pressure by grasping the wrists and holding exerciser's fists apart.

Butterfly—Exerciser starts with arms straight and at the sides. Partner, from the back, attempts to hold the arms down while exerciser lifts straight arms to the sides. With arms above the head (partner holding) try to move them down to the sides.

Back Builder—Exerciser spreads the legs and bends forward at the waist with head up. Partner faces exerciser and places hands on the back of exerciser's shoulders. Exerciser attempts to stand upright while partner pushes down.

Push-up with Resistance—Exerciser is in push-up position with arms bent, so that the body is about halfway up from the floor. Partner straddles or stands alongside exerciser's head and puts pressure on the top of the shoulders by pushing down. The amount of pressure takes judgment by the partner. Too much pressure causes the exerciser to collapse.

MATERIALS ORDER FORM

FITNESSGRAM

With the initial order of computer cards the agency will receive FREE FITNESSGRAM System Software, Test Administration Manual, and Computer Reference Manual per box of cards ordered.

		QTY	UNIT PRICE	AMOUNT DUE
Box of 200 Computer Cards	02101		$22.00	
Box of 600 Computer Cards	02102		$60.00	
Box 200 Non-computer Cards	02103		$26.00	
Box 600 Non-computer Cards	02104		$78.00	
Individual Non-computer Card	02105		$0.15	
Special Enrollment Package	02111		$76.00	
Includes 600 cards, FREE software and Computer Reference Manual, Test Administration Manual, calipers, Pacer tape an lap counter, curl-up measuring strips, Teachers's Sample Kit				
COMPUTER MATERIALS				
IBM Computer Manual	02201		$10.00	
Mac Computer Manual	02202		$10.00	
II Computer Manual	02203		$10.00	
Non-computer Manual	02205		$8.00	
Test Administration Manual	02206		$10.00	
IBM Software	02211		$6.00	
Mac Software	02212		$6.00	
IIe Software	02213		$6.00	
IIgs Software	02214		$6.00	
SUPPORT MATERIALS				
Curl-up Strips (specify grade)	02301		$0.45	
Clipboard	02302		$7.99	
Calipers	02303		$4.75	
Pacer Tape and Lap Counter	02304		$10.00	
Awards Sample Kit	02306		$9.50	
IT'S YOUR MOVE MATERIALS				
IYM Hip Hopper Set of 35 Booklets (K-2)	02401		$19.55	
IYM Move & Shaker Set of 35 Booklets (3-4)	02402		$19.55	
IYM Slam Jammer Set of 35 Booklet (5-6)	02403		$19.55	
IYM Hip Hopper Button (K-2) each	02404		$0.35	
IYM Mover & Shaker Button (3-4) each	02405		$0.35	
IYM Slam Jammer Button (5-6) each	02406		$0.35	
GET FIT ITEMS				
Certificate GF	02501		$0.25	
Emblem GF	02502		$1.15	
Poster	02503		$1.60	
Ribbon 1st GF	02504		$0.25	
Ribbon 2nd GF	02505		$0.25	
Ribbon 3rd GF	02506		$0.25	
Ribbon 4th GF	02507		$0.25	
Button GF	02508		$0.35	
I'M FIT ITEMS				
Pencil IF	02601		$0.15	
Emblem IF	02602		$1.15	
Sticker Sheet IF	02603		$0.35	
Ribbon 1st IF	02604		$0.25	
Ribbon 2nd IF	02605		$0.25	
Ribbon 3rd IF	02606		$0.25	
Ribbon 4th IF	02607		$0.25	
Button IF	02608		$0.35	
HONOR AND FIT FOR LIFE ITEMS				
Honor Certificate	02701		$0.45	
FFL Certificate	02703		$0.25	
FFL Ruler	02704		$1.00	
INSTRUCTOR ITEMS				
T-shirts	02801-05		$6.00	
Tyvek Jackets	02810-14		$27.50	

SUB TOTAL _____

Transfer sub total and complete ordering information on reverse side.

HOW TO ORDER:
Be sure to provide all requested information. *Do not send cash or postage stamps.*

PHONE ORDERS:
Call AAHPERD Sales 1(800) 321-0789 or FITNESSGRAM Sales 1(800) 635-7050. Institutional purchase order ($50 minimum) or Visa/Mastercard ($10.00 minimum) required. Shipping and handling charges will be added to your order.

MAIL ORDERS:
Order must be accompanied by payment or official purchase order ($50.00 minimum). Shipping and handling charges will be billed.

METHOD OF PAYMENT:
(Note: Foreign orders must be prepaid in U.S. currency.) If paying by check please include shipping and handling charges. Shipping and handling will be billed on all orders charged to institutional PO or Visa/Mastercard. Please check the appropriate box:
☐ Check or money order enclosed
☐ Purchase order ($50.00 Minimum)
☐ Visa ☐ Mastercard ($10.00 Minimum)
Please include shipping and handling charges as shown in the chart below.

Print Card Number Clearly

Visa is 13 numbers; Mastercard is 16 numbers

Expiration Date: _____

Signature: _____

Purchase Order #: _____
($50.00 Minimum)

SHIPPING/HANDLING FEES:
Each box of 200 FITNESSGRAM cards $4.50
Each box of 600 FITNESSGRAM cards $7.00
All other items based on amount purchased.

	Continental US	Foreign Orders
0 - $24.99	$5.25	$11.75
$25.00-$49.99	$7.50	19.25
$50.00-$99.99	$9.50	25.00
$100+	10% of Total Order	25% of Total Order

*Shipping/handling charges will be billed for phone, charge, and institutional PO orders. Domestic orders shipped UPS. Foreign orders shipped Surface Mail.

RUSH ORDERS
FLAT Order Charge $25.00 Next Day

*If only one item in a multiple RUSH order is available, it will be keyed as two separate orders; the rush order will receive the $25.00 shipping charge, and the second will receive regular ground.

COMPUTER INFORMATION
Please provide required software specifications.
Check one software type:
☐ DOS ☐ Windows ☐ Macintosh
☐ IIe ☐ IIgs-1 drive ☐ IIgs-2 drives
Check disk size: ☐ 5.25" disks ☐ 3.5" disks

MATERIALS ORDER FORM

MATERIALS FOR INSTRUCTION		QTY	UNIT PRICE	AMOUNT DUE
Educational Kit (K-6) & Instructor's Guide	246-28570		$37.95	
Educational Kit (6-12) & Instructor's Guide	246-28576		$37.95	
Instructor's Comprehensive Guide	0-88314-452-2		$6.95	
Flextester	242-27708		$74.95	
Physical Best Skinfold Caliper	242-27206		$10.00	
Skinfold Video	242-28332		$29.95	
Activity Logs (30 per pack)	246-28616		$5.00	
Contracts (30 per pack)	246-28618		$5.00	
Report Cards (30 per pack)	246-28620		$3.50	
Physical Best Wall Chart	246-28684		$10.00	
Video: PB: Integrating Concepts w/Activities Gr. K-6	246-28934		$19.95	
Video: PB: Integrating Concepts w/Activities Gr. 6-12	246-28936		$19.95	
CERTIFICATES				
Fitness Activity Certificate	246-28676		$0.35	
Fitness Goals Certificate	246-28678		$0.35	
Health Fitness Certificate	246-28680		$0.35	
BADGES K-12				
Fitness Activity Badge K-12	246-28734		$0.75	
Fitness Goal Badge K-12	246-28736		$0.75	
Health Fitness Badge Kindergarten	246-28738		$0.75	
Health Fitness Badge 1	246-28740		$0.75	
Health Fitness Badge 2	246-28742		$0.75	
Health Fitness Badge 3	246-28744		$0.75	
Health Fitness Badge 4	246-28746		$0.75	
Health Fitness Badge 5	246-28748		$0.75	
Health Fitness Badge 6	246-28750		$0.75	
Health Fitness Badge 7	246-28752		$0.75	
Health Fitness Badge 8	246-28754		$0.75	
Health Fitness Badge 9	246-28756		$0.75	
Health Fitness Badge 10	246-28758		$0.75	
Health Fitness Badge 11	246-28760		$0.75	
Health Fitness Badge 12	246-28762		$0.75	
SHIRTS				
Physical Best T Shirt Small	246-28490		$10.00	
Physical Best T Shirt Medium	246-28492		$10.00	
Physical Best T Shirt Large	246-28494		$10.00	
Physical Best T Shirt X Large	246-28496		$10.00	
Physical Best T Shirt XX Large	246-28914		$10.00	
MISCELLANEOUS				
Shoelaces (pair)	246-28916		$2.00	
Pencils (25 per pack)	246-28918		$5.00	
Stickers (25 per pack)	246-28920		$2.00	
Lapel Pins	246-28922		$4.00	

BILL TO:

Company or school

Address

City   State   Zip

SHIP TO:

Company or school

Address

City   State   Zip

CONTACT PERSON:

School District

School Building

Contact Name

Address

City   State   Zip

Phone #

Order by FAX

**AAHPERD FAX
(301) 567-9553**

**FITNESSGRAM FAX
(214) 991-4626**

SUB TOTAL _____

SUB TOTAL FROM PAGE 1 _____

SHIPPING/HANDLING _____

TX add 8.25%, VA add 4.5%, MD add 5% TAX _____

TOTAL _____

PRICES SUBJECT TO CHANGE WITHOUT NOTICE!

MAIL THIS ORDER FORM TO:
AAHPERD Publications
P.O. Box 385, Oxen Hill, MD 20750-0385
or
The Prudential FITNESSGRAM
The Cooper Institute for Aerobics Research
12330 Preston Road, Dallas, TX 75230

PLEASE ALLOW 2-4 WEEKS FOR DELIVERY • NO RETURNS ACCEPTED ON AAHPERD PRODUCTS